PATIENTS' PREFERENCES MATTER
Stop the silent misdiagnosis

Al Mulley, Chris Trimble, Glyn Elwyn

To Paul, with great regard for all you have done to improve health care and health for all!

Cal

The King's Fund>

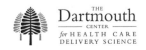

THE
Dartmouth
CENTER
for HEALTH CARE
DELIVERY SCIENCE

The King's Fund seeks to understand how the health system in England can be improved. Using that insight, we help to shape policy, transform services and bring about behaviour change. Our work includes research, analysis, leadership development and service improvement. We also offer a wide range of resources to help everyone working in health to share knowledge, learning and ideas.

Published by

The King's Fund

11-13 Cavendish Square

London W1G 0AN

Tel: 020 7307 2568

Fax: 020 7307 2801

www.kingsfund.org.uk

© The King's Fund 2012

First published 2012 by The King's Fund

Charity registration number: 1126980

ISBN: 978 1 85717 637 7

A catalogue record for this publication is available from the British Library

Available from:

The King's Fund

11-13 Cavendish Square

London W1G 0AN

Tel: 020 7307 2568

Fax: 020 7307 2801

Email: publications@kingsfund.org.uk

www.kingsfund.org.uk/publications

Edited by Kathryn O'Neill

Typeset by Peter Powell Origination & Print Limited

Printed in the UK by The King's Fund

Contents

About the authors

Al Mulley is Director of The Dartmouth Center for Health Care Delivery Science and Professor of Medicine at Dartmouth. He was awarded a Bachelor of Arts degree from Dartmouth in 1970, followed by Doctor of Medicine and Master of Public Policy degrees from Harvard Medical School and the Kennedy School of Government in 1975. Before returning to Dartmouth in 2010, he spent 35 years on the Harvard faculty at Massachusetts General Hospital, where he was the founding Chief of the General Medicine Division and Director of the Medical Practices Evaluation Center. He is co-editor of the leading text *Primary Care Medicine,* now in its eighth edition. Together with Jack Wennberg, Al was a founding director of the Informed Medical Decisions Foundation, where he continues to serve as senior clinical adviser. He has served as a visiting professor and consultant to government agencies, health care organisations and academic medical centres in North America, Europe, Asia and Africa. Al has worked with the NHS in a number of capacities over the past two decades. In 2010, he was appointed to the Health Foundation's Improvement Science Network. In 2011, he was named the first International Visiting Fellow at The King's Fund in London, and International Consultant to the Chinese Hospital Association.

Chris Trimble is Adjunct Professor of Business Administration at The Dartmouth Center for Health Care Delivery Science and at the Tuck School of Business at Dartmouth. He holds a Masters in Business Administration degree from Tuck and a Bachelor of Science degree from the University of Virginia. Chris has dedicated more than 10 years to studying a single challenge that vexes even the best-managed organisations: how to execute an innovation initiative. He is co-author of four books on the topic, including *The Other Side of Innovation: Solving the execution challenge,* with Vijay Govindarajan. Chris's career mixes academic research with practical application. He has advised dozens of organisations and has delivered speeches and workshops all over the world. Chris is currently immersed in an effort to apply his work to the specific challenge of innovation in health care delivery.

Glyn Elwyn is a physician-researcher, currently Visiting Professor and Senior Scientist at The Dartmouth Center for Health Care Delivery Science and The Dartmouth Institute for Health Policy and Clinical Practice, Dartmouth College. He also holds the following positions: Distinguished Research Chair at Cardiff University and, in the Netherlands, Visiting Chair at the Scientific Institute for Quality of Healthcare, Radboud University Nijmegen Medical Centre, and the University of Maastricht. After completing a Bachelor of Arts degree, he qualified in medicine, leading innovative primary care developments in the UK.

He completed a Masters in Medical Education and a Doctorate under the guidance of Richard Grol in the Netherlands. He leads interdisciplinary research teams that deploy a range of investigative methods. His research examines the implementation of shared decision-making, user-centred design of patient decision support, and the integration of these into routine health care. His current focus is on the development, use and evaluation of option grids. He has published 231 peer-reviewed articles and is co-editor of *Shared Decision-Making in Health Care: Achieving evidence-based patient choice* (Oxford University Press, 2nd ed 2009).

Foreword

When I arrived at The King's Fund in 2010, one of my ambitions was to bring a stronger international focus to the Fund's work. I was therefore delighted when Al Mulley, then at Harvard and now at Dartmouth, accepted our invitation to be the Fund's first international visiting fellow.

I first met Al in 1987 at an international conference on health care variations held in Copenhagen where he was speaking on a platform that included Jack Wennberg and Klim McPherson. Al spoke about the history of research into variations, citing Glover's seminal work in England and emphasising the need to base treatment decisions on patient preferences as well as professional judgement. Al's ability to apply evidence to important and difficult issues in health care in a way that pointed to practical solutions marked him out as an influential figure in health services research.

We renewed contact a decade ago when I worked in the Department of Health and invited Al to lead an expert seminar on shared decision-making. His contribution helped to inform the then government's policy on patient choice, taking the argument about choice beyond the narrow confines of choice of practice or hospital into the much more important and challenging area of choice of treatment. By that stage Al was testing out ways of engaging patients in shared decision-making, marking an important transition in the application of theory into practice.

The fact that this paper returns to arguments I first heard articulated 25 years ago speaks volumes about the time it takes to get changes in the relationship between patients and health care professionals accepted and implemented. Together with his fellow authors, Al makes a persuasive case as to why 'no decision about me without me' is much more than a sound bite or an empty political slogan. Only by understanding patient preferences and incorporating them into treatment decisions will it be possible to reduce unwarranted variations and deliver appropriate care.

After the sound and fury that accompanied debate on the Health and Social Care Bill, it is refreshing to be able to focus on issues that really make a difference to patients and their care. The King's Fund's work in 2012 and beyond will continue to emphasise the opportunities to improve the experience of patients and the quality of care as the NHS reforms are translated from the statute book into change on the ground. The time to stop the silent misdiagnosis is now and the need is urgent.

The Fund is delighted to be publishing this paper and hope it will be widely read and acted on. Its findings are timely and relevant to all who have the best interests of the patient at heart. Implementing the ideas set out here would be an important step in transforming the role of patients in the NHS from passive users into active and engaged partners in care.

Chris Ham
Chief Executive

May 2012

Acknowledgements

The authors are grateful to The King's Fund, and to Chris Ham and Anna Dixon in particular, for making it possible for one of us, Al Mulley, to join the organisation as its first International Visiting Fellow. Thanks to this Fellowship, we had access to the deep expertise of the Fund's staff, as well as many people in the Fund's network who generously volunteered their time for open-ended discussions when this paper was in its formative stages. We would also like to thank those who carefully reviewed drafts, including Michael Barry, Aileen Clarke, Phil DaSilva, Anna Dixon, Jack Fowler, Chris Ham, Bob Hansen, Patrick Lee, Ben Moulton, Karen Sepucha, Jonathan Skinner, and Anne Winter.

Competing interests

Al Mulley is senior clinical adviser to the Informed Medical Decisions Foundation and receives consulting fees for decision aid content and design. He also receives royalties from Health Dialog, which distributes decision aids and other forms of decision support developed in collaboration with the Foundation.

Chris Trimble is an author and consultant on the topic of innovation and implementation. His research is currently funded through The Dartmouth Center for Health Care Delivery Science.

Glyn Elwyn is the instigator of the Option Grid Collaborative, which develops tools to support shared decision-making. These tools are freely available using a Creative Commons licence. His research has been supported by grants from the Informed Medical Decisions Foundation, as well as travel and speaking fees. He holds research grants from the Health Foundation and the BUPA Foundation. He is a Director of Prepared to Share, a training consultancy for shared decision-making, and is an adviser to Emmi Solutions in the United States.

Executive summary

Many doctors aspire to excellence in diagnosing disease. Far fewer, unfortunately, aspire to the same standards of excellence in diagnosing what patients want. In fact, we will present an accumulation of evidence which shows that preference misdiagnoses are commonplace. In part, this is because doctors are rarely made aware that they have made a preference misdiagnosis. It is the silent misdiagnosis.

The NHS must break this silence. It must stop the silent misdiagnosis. When it does so, it will score three distinct victories. First, patients, who can suffer just as much from a preference misdiagnosis as a medical misdiagnosis, will get the medicine they would choose were they well informed – that is, if they had better information about treatment options, outcomes, and evidence. Second, the NHS's aspiration to create an 'internal market' will finally have a chance to achieve its full potential. Third, because patients choose fewer treatments when fully informed, the NHS could save billions of pounds.

The problem of the silent misdiagnosis is widespread. Several studies show that patients choose different treatments after they become better informed. In addition, there are wide gaps between what patients want and what doctors *think* patients want. Finally, there are dramatic geographic variations in care that can only partially be explained by causes other than the silent misdiagnosis.

The most important step the NHS must take in order to stop the silent misdiagnosis is conceptually straightforward: it must measure and report the incidence of preference misdiagnoses. It must also challenge a handful of entrenched but erroneous assumptions that are inconsistent with the mindset necessary to tackle the problem of the silent misdiagnosis. Those assumptions are: (1) that science alone determines need, (2) that variation in care is the problem, (3) that patient choice is about time and location, (4) that 'the market' can sort out health care, and (5) that commissioners can calculate need.

Furthermore, the NHS must support doctors in their efforts to make more accurate preference diagnoses. It must do so by providing doctors with more and better information about what patients want, and by providing patients with more and better information about options, outcomes, and evidence. To assess progress, the NHS should implement measures that indicate how much doctors and patients have learned.

To fully realise the agenda that we propose here, the NHS must recognise the need for new, dedicated teams focused on gathering and disseminating information. It must also aid commissioners in shifting their focus, from trying to calculate need to trying to eliminate preference misdiagnoses, so that patients receive the care they need (and no less), and the care they want (and no more).

The problem of the silent misdiagnosis

When Linda was diagnosed with breast cancer, she was devastated. She was 58. She quickly found support from others who had dealt with breast cancer. Nonetheless, her anxieties as she awaited surgery nearly overwhelmed her.

Linda's operation went well. However, when the pathologist examined Linda's excised breast tissue, he could find no signs of cancer. It turned out that Linda had been healthy all along. She had been misdiagnosed.

When the hospital's medical director was informed of the misdiagnosis, he immediately set in motion a thorough investigation. Before long, it was clear what happened. There had been an administrative mix-up in handling the results of the needle biopsy of Linda's breast lump. The staff responsible for the error were identified and called to account. The hospital launched immediate corrective actions to try to eliminate similar errors. Linda, for her part, considered taking legal action.

When Susan was diagnosed with breast cancer, she was more stoical than Linda. She was 78, other members of her family had had breast cancer, and she had already been treated for a serious illness – heart failure. She dreaded having surgery, but her surgeon was insistent.

Susan's mastectomy was also routine, and in her case the pathologist's report quickly confirmed the diagnosis. There was clear evidence of cancer in her breast tissue, and the surgery had been successful in removing it.

Nonetheless, Susan struggled after surgery. She felt anxiety and sadness. She felt less than she once was. Making matters worse, Susan spoke to a friend of the same age who had been diagnosed with breast cancer but had opted *not* to have surgery. The friend's logic was simple. She reckoned that if she simply slowed the cancer's advance with hormone therapy, then it was likely that she'd die of something else before the breast cancer had any adverse effect.

After the conversation, the emotion Susan felt most intensely was regret. Knowing that her decision could not be reversed, she tried not to dwell on it, and she never spoke of it again. The truth, however, was that had Susan been aware of all her options and the available evidence in advance, she would not have proceeded with the surgery.

Linda and Susan were both victims of misdiagnoses. Linda's was the more recognisable medical misdiagnosis, while Susan's was a more subtle *preference misdiagnosis*. Susan's doctor did not accurately determine the treatment that Susan would have chosen were she fully informed.

While the two misdiagnoses were distinct in nature, both patients suffered similarly. Both endured the needless trauma of breast surgery. The scalpels were equally sharp, and their recoveries were equally fraught.

The stories differ, however, in the response to the misdiagnosis. In Linda's case, the corrective actions were numerous, immediate, and loud. For Susan, there were no corrective actions at all. The problem was not even recognised as a problem. Susan's was a silent misdiagnosis.

Recognising the full challenge of diagnosis

For many doctors, the spectre of a misdiagnosis or a missed diagnosis can provoke sleepless nights. An untreated disease can progress to the point that it becomes untreatable, while a treated non-disease can also harm patients to a greater or lesser extent. Furthermore, diagnostic errors cut right to the core of a doctor's self-image and self-esteem. They are also the most common reason why doctors get sued (Weingart *et al* 2000).

As such, most doctors are willing to expend tremendous personal energy, not to mention institutional resources, to avoid a misdiagnosis. They order laboratory tests and images. They call on specialists and subspecialists. They rely on years of medical training, all backed by an enormous volume of scientific research, to ensure that the diagnosis is right. The mindset is straightforward: get the diagnosis right, and you get the treatment right. Treatment is a function of diagnosis. It can be expressed as a simple equation:

$$T = f(D)$$

However, for all of the effort that the medical profession puts into getting the diagnosis right, diagnostic efforts generally proceed in ignorance of a crucial variable in the diagnostic equation: patient preferences. A better equation would be:

$$T = f(D_M, D_P)$$

… where D_M is the medical diagnosis and D_P is the preference diagnosis. We define a preference diagnosis as a doctor's inference of what a patient would choose if he or she were fully informed. It is an *inference* because no patient – save perhaps the patient who is also a doctor and world-renowned specialist in the very disease with which he or she is afflicted – is *fully* informed. Preference diagnosis, like medical diagnosis, is often a best estimate based on imperfect information.

For many doctors, the addition of a preference diagnosis seems, at first glance, a trivial amendment. Their intuition is supported by two assumptions; but both, as it turns out, are misguided. The first assumption is that the medical diagnosis must be, by far, the dominant of the two factors. This is just not so. In fact, for much of modern medical care, the right treatment is also dependent on patient preferences (Eddy 1994; Wennberg 2004). Indeed, a presumption that the medical diagnosis and the preference diagnosis are of equal importance is closer to the truth. Furthermore, the consequences of preference misdiagnoses are anything but trivial. As Susan's and Linda's stories show, the consequence of an error in preference diagnosis can be every bit as serious as the consequences of an error in medical diagnosis.

The second erroneous assumption is that diagnosing a patient's preferences is simple and straightforward. It is little wonder that doctors hold this belief; entry into the profession demands years of training, and a great deal of it focuses on medical diagnosis. But little, if any of it, focuses on preference diagnosis – the frequent talk of 'patient-centred medicine' notwithstanding. Doctors are taught that making an accurate medical diagnosis can be devilishly challenging. It is a task worthy of highly trained professionals, sophisticated laboratory equipment, and the full arsenal of medical science. But what of diagnosing preferences? Is it really any more complicated than getting to know your patient a little?

The answer is yes, it is substantially more complicated than that. Nonetheless, most doctors believe that they are already quite good at diagnosing patient preferences. They are not just misguided in their self-assessment, they are dangerously wrong. Indeed, there are breathtaking gaps between what patients want and what doctors *think* they want. For example, doctors believe that 71 per cent of patients with breast cancer rate keeping their breast as a top priority. But what is the actual figure reported by patients? 7 per cent (Lee *et al* 2010). Furthermore, doctors believe that 96 per cent of breast cancer patients considering chemotherapy rate living as long as possible a top priority. But what is the actual figure reported by patients? 59 per cent (Lee *et al* 2010).

These are just two examples of data from an accumulation of evidence which shows that doctors, in general, are unskilled at diagnosing what patients want. (Much more evidence will be presented in a later section of this paper.) How could such a dreadful state of affairs persist?

It certainly could not persist in other professions. Consider business. When an executive fails to understand what his or her customers want, the consequences are severe – bankruptcy, for example. As such, business professionals take the challenge of diagnosing customer wants and needs with an intensity that is deadly serious – especially when customers are not fully aware of what they want, or unable to clearly articulate it. They employ a wide range of tools and techniques.

They call on outside experts who specialise in nothing other than figuring out what customers want. They bring to bear sophisticated quantitative and qualitative analyses, all backed by a vast array of academic research.

As a result, in a business setting, presenting data that show an enormous gap between what customers want and what an executive team believes its customers want is tantamount to accusing the team of incompetence. When similar data are presented to a room full of doctors, however, it barely creates a ripple. Perhaps this is because doctors believe that patients are too uninformed to know what is good for them, or perhaps it is because the importance of diagnosing preferences gets inadequate attention in medical training.

Whatever the reason, doctors simply do not view diagnosing patient preferences as an important part of their work. This incongruous state of affairs persists for one simple reason: doctors rarely face serious consequences – not bankruptcy, not malpractice claims, not anything – from a preference misdiagnosis. It is the silent misdiagnosis.

Our central recommendation: measure the accuracy of preference diagnoses

The NHS must break the silence. It must do so by implementing measures and publishing data – loudly – on the accuracy of preference diagnoses.

As any magazine editor who has ever published a ranking is well aware, the mere existence of widely published data galvanises action. In time, the buzz at any gathering of doctors could be just as likely to focus on skill in figuring out what well-informed patients want as it is to focus on the complexities of disease or the latest advances in treatment. Individual doctors could take as much pride in accurately diagnosing patient preferences as they do in accurately diagnosing disease. Stories like Susan's could become rare.

Individual doctors, however, should not be expected to bear the full burden of the challenge of improving the accuracy of preference diagnoses. Doing so takes a commitment of time, energy, tools, and special training that is well beyond the resource base currently available to individual doctors. Addressing the problem will require a co-ordinated effort that involves multiple levels of the NHS, including patients, frontline clinicians, medical directors, commissioners, senior executives, and policy-makers.

The pay-off: a cascade of wins for the NHS

The silent misdiagnosis is a quiet problem with high-decibel implications. Putting a stop to it will lead to at least three distinct and powerful victories: in ethics, policy, and finance.

Delivering the right treatment, every time

Let's start with the obvious. Operating on a patient who wouldn't want the operation if they were fully informed is as ethically dubious as anything that happens in medicine (Elwyn *et al* 2012). The fact that the silent misdiagnosis is hard to see does not justify ignoring it. Indeed, ethics is quite often about what you do when nobody is watching.

Patients deserve better. They deserve to be treated with dignity. They deserve an NHS that is deeply vigilant about respecting each patient's preferences.

Furthermore, stopping the silent misdiagnosis will leave clinicians feeling better about their work and better about their profession. Indeed, top performers in most professions generally experience a burst of renewed energy when they discover new ways to achieve higher levels of excellence.

Medicine is a field rich in intrinsic rewards, but those rewards can be redoubled if doctors can be confident that they are delivering the care that patients would want if they were fully informed. Indeed, few clinicians would feel good about delivering an unwanted treatment, were they aware that it was happening. Similarly, few clinicians would feel good about *failing* to deliver a treatment that *would* meet a patient's preferences, were they aware that it was happening.

Addressing a longstanding problem in health policy

Beyond its ethical dimension, the silent misdiagnosis represents a fundamental flaw in the essential logic that underpins the health policies pursued by the NHS for more than two decades. In 1989, Kenneth Clarke, the then Health Secretary, initiated the creation of an internal market within the NHS. This led to the NHS we have today, and its most controversial characteristic – the split between providers and purchasers, between supply and demand.

The American economist Alain Enthoven heavily influenced Clarke's thinking (Enthoven 1985). Enthoven studied the NHS in the mid-1980s as the storm clouds of a deep budgetary crisis gathered. His assessment was that the NHS was gridlocked in resistance to change. Doctors jealously guarded their autonomy, and they guarded it well because they had all the power. They routinely strengthened their lock on the allegiance of patients and the public by blaming managers and politicians for withholding resources and thus denying services. So heavily empowered, doctors had too little incentive for innovation, service redesign, or clinical improvement.

Enthoven's central recommendation was to subject doctors to market forces. He had much more confidence in Adam Smith's invisible hand than he did in a restructured organisational chart. But he was far from fundamentalist in his thinking. He understood that market mechanisms are imperfect, particularly in health care. His vision was not for an unrestrained market romp; rather, it was for a carefully managed market. As such, his specific recommendations were many. Of particular importance, he asked, pointedly, 'How will general managers measure patient preferences and inject them into decision-making?'.

Enthoven understood that markets function as described in introductory economics textbooks only when there is perfect information – that is, both buyers and sellers understand exactly what they are transacting. And he knew that it would be hard to identify an industry further from this textbook ideal than health care. Doctors know far more than patients; they are the ones with years of medical training, the ability to order sophisticated tests, and access to the latest research. The average patient, by contrast, not only has no medical training, but has also been conditioned to believe simply that 'the doctor knows best'.

This was not the market that Adam Smith visualised. He lived in a world of bakers and candlestick makers, not pathologists and oncologists.

Enthoven's recommendations were nuanced, but nuance is often a casualty of politics. The received wisdom, and the one that took hold under Kenneth Clarke, was that an internal market could turn the NHS around. Indeed, the NHS and the Community Care Act, which set the changes in motion, did little to specify how the internal market would be guided or regulated. As a result, health authorities operated with little useful information to guide their purchasing decisions. They had no mechanism to assess what patients would want were they fully informed, and thus no sense of true demand for services.

This situation persists to this day. Commissioners make purchasing decisions with little ability to assess true demand. Until the NHS stops the silent misdiagnosis, commissioners will remain blind, the internal market will remain perilously flawed, and the foundation upon which the UK's health policy rests will remain flimsy.

Solving the budget crisis

By stopping the silent misdiagnosis, the NHS could also make considerable progress in tackling its ailing finances. The government currently projects an astonishing £20 billion shortfall in NHS funding by 2014, which amounts roughly to 17 per cent of the NHS's projected budget. There are two possible outcomes. Either the NHS will figure out how to increase its productivity by 3–4 per cent a year – the so-called Nicholson challenge – or it will be forced into draconian cuts that would reduce quality of care. Waiting times will get longer, and the public will be anything but silent.

A sense of resignation could easily take hold. To our knowledge, no health system – anywhere in the world, at any point in history – has ever achieved 3–4 per cent productivity gains per year. Nonetheless, such gains are possible. Indeed, the NHS's finest hour could be near at hand, because a major component of the solution is as simple in principle as it is counterintuitive: *give patients what they would want were they fully informed.*

Health care may be the only industry in which giving customers what they really want would save money. Well-informed patients consume less medicine – and not just a little bit less, but much less. When doctors accurately diagnose patient preferences, an enormous source of waste – the delivery of unwanted services – is eliminated. It is particularly notable that when doctors accurately diagnose the preferences of patients struggling with long-term conditions, those patients are far more likely to keep their conditions under control, leading to fewer hospitalisations and emergency department visits (Wennberg and Marr 2010).

The 2002 Wanless Report estimated the potential annual savings at £30 billion, or 16 per cent of the projected budget by 2022 (Wanless 2002). That estimate was based on an optimistic scenario of maximum patient engagement, but we believe nonetheless that the potential financial gain from stopping the silent misdiagnosis is comparable in magnitude to the potential financial gain from improved adherence to evidence-based clinical guidelines. Indeed, the two together could bridge the entire budget shortfall, and both opportunities should be pursued. As yet, however, the NHS has acted only on the latter opportunity, through the creation, in 1999, of the National Institute for Health and Clinical Excellence (NICE) and its practice guidelines.

The politics of health care finance can be tense and exhausting. The source of much of the conflict, however, is the instinct that whatever the solution, there will be winners and losers. A move to stop the silent misdiagnosis, however, is not a win–lose prospect. The major constituents all win: it is a win for patients, who get what they would want were they fully informed; it is a win for the general public, as national resources are redirected to investments in education, infrastructure, and more; and it is a win for the health profession. Doctors become more confident that they deliver the right services every time, and experience less in the way of oppressive pressures for ever-improved operational efficiency. All of this is possible if the NHS can stop the silent misdiagnosis.

This paper will continue with four additional major sections. In the first, we lay out the specific evidence that demonstrates the magnitude of the silent misdiagnosis. In the second, we describe the essential actions that the NHS must take organisation-wide, especially measuring and widely reporting the accuracy of preference diagnoses. In the third, we outline several possible innovation initiatives that could increase the accuracy of preference diagnoses. Finally, we outline a framework for implementation of the changes we recommend.

The evidence

Misdiagnosis of patient preferences is commonplace within the NHS and in health services around the world. We frame our discussion of the evidence that supports this conclusion with the diagram and brief discussion of key terms below.

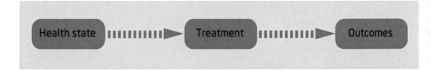

We will be discussing *health states, treatments*, and *outcomes*. Typically, doctors make a medical diagnosis to determine the patient's health state. Having done so, the doctor and patient choose a treatment in anticipation of achieving a desirable outcome.

In discussing treatment options with a doctor, a patient might express one or both of two types of preference – either a *treatment preference* or an *outcome preference*. Either is a valuable indicator as the doctor makes a *preference diagnosis*. Again, a preference diagnosis is the doctor's inference of the treatment the patient would choose if they were fully informed.

When a patient clearly expresses a treatment preference, it is a strong indicator of the right preference diagnosis, but it is not necessarily conclusive. Only very rarely is a patient *fully* informed. A doctor, for example, might reasonably say 'I hear you making a very clear treatment choice, but it is a very important choice you are making, and I am not honestly sure if you fully understand the implications of your choice' and continue to engage the patient in further discussion.

As a general rule, patients express outcome preferences more easily than treatment preferences. Also, as a general rule, as patients become more informed, they become more likely to express a treatment preference. In some cases, the cause–effect relationship between treatment and outcome is so intuitive and obvious that the distinction vanishes. For example, if a patient opts for the treatment of a mastectomy, the most immediate outcome will be living without a breast. In other cases, patients may shy away from expressing a treatment preference. The treatment options may be sufficiently difficult to understand or so heavily laden with uncertainty that the patient can comfortably express only an outcome preference. These patients defer the treatment choice to the person they view as their expert adviser – their doctor.

There are three categories of evidence which support the conclusion that the silent misdiagnosis is widespread:

- *Studies of treatment preferences.* These studies show how treatment preferences change after patients become well informed.

- *Studies of outcome preferences.* These studies show differences between the outcomes that patients prefer and the outcomes that doctors *think* they prefer.

- *Studies of geographic variations in care.* There are dramatic variations in care between geographic regions. These variations can only be partially explained by causes other than the silent misdiagnosis.

Patients make different choices when well informed

Several researchers have shown that treatment decisions change – sometimes dramatically – after populations of patients become well informed. This is the category of evidence that offers the clearest and most direct indication of the silent misdiagnosis.

For example, an international Cochrane Review that included 11 trials involving major elective surgeries showed that demand declined by 20 per cent after patients became well informed. This systematic review reported consistent evidence that as patients became better informed, they made different decisions and felt more confident (Stacey *et al* 2011). These results might be even more dramatic if clinicians were more skilled in diagnosing preferences.

In addition, consider the following studies of single conditions.

- *Benign prostate disease.* Patients typically seek treatment because of urinary symptoms. Surgery can ameliorate these symptoms, but there is a trade-off. Many patients suffer from a form of post-surgical sexual dysfunction. An observational study showed that when patients were well informed about the trade-off, 40 per cent fewer preferred surgery (Wagner *et al* 1995) – *40 per cent!*[1]

Surgeons had systematically and dramatically overestimated patients' preference for symptom relief and underestimated their preference to avoid sexual dysfunction. Indeed, this simple intervention – informing patients of the available evidence regarding the outcomes of treatment – reduced the incidence of surgery to a rate that was lower than all but one of 306 hospital referral regions in the United States (Dartmouth Atlas of Health Care 2012).

---

1 A subsequent randomised trial showed the same 40 per cent reduction, though the sample size was too small for the results to be statistically significant (Barry *et al* 1997). A later trial in the UK showed an increase in the proportion choosing surgery, but that trial was also too small to be significant (Murray *et al* 2001).

■ *Abnormal bleeding from the uterus.* When women with abnormal bleeding from the uterus seek treatment, they may be offered one of a number of treatments, ranging from surgical removal of the uterus to simply waiting until menopause. A British randomised trial showed a relative reduction in the rate of surgery of more than 20 per cent (an absolute decline of 10 per cent, from 48 per cent to 38 per cent) when women were informed with a decision aid and interviewed to clarify their treatment preferences (Kennedy *et al* 2002).

■ *Coronary heart disease.* A randomised trial of a decision aid in Toronto showed a relative reduction in preference for surgical treatment (with coronary artery bypass graft surgery or percutaneous coronary intervention) of more than 20 per cent (a decrease from 75 per cent to 58 per cent) for patients with chest pain diagnosed as stable angina. This is an even more stunning number when put in context. The per capita surgical rate in Toronto was already quite low – just half of New York's rate and one-third of the rate in other parts of the United States (Morgan *et al* 2000). At a population level, the new rate was lower than that of *all* of the 306 hospital referral regions in the United States.

How could this happen? Most patients with this medical diagnosis believed that bypassing or opening a clogged coronary artery would reduce the risk of a heart attack; but it doesn't. Being better informed changed their preferences. The same avoidable ignorance is equally prevalent today: 88 per cent of patients still have the same misperception, despite definitive evidence to the contrary published in 2007(Boden *et al* 2007; Rothberg *et al* 2010).

■ *Back pain.* In a study of back pain, patients with herniated discs were more than 30 per cent *less* likely to choose surgery (a decrease from 47 per cent to 32 per cent) when fully informed, while those with spinal stenosis were more than 30 per cent *more* likely to choose surgery (an increase from 29 per cent to 39 per cent) (Deyo *et al* 2000). Given the data on outcomes, this bidirectional result was not surprising. The evidence shows that patients with herniated discs are likely to get better eventually even without surgery, while those with spinal stenosis are not. When patients understood the evidence, their decisions changed.

Note that it is the magnitude of change, not the direction of change, that indicates the incidence of the silent misdiagnosis. Indeed, the primary reason to stop the silent misdiagnosis is not to cut costs, but to ensure that each patient gets the care that they would choose if they were fully informed – no less and no more. Thankfully, far more studies show a decrease rather than an increase in consumption of services. Though the potential reduction in health care expenditures is a secondary effect, it is, of course, welcome.

In a similar study in Canada, expert physicians were asked to identify candidates for joint replacement based only on medical information (that is, excluding patient preferences). Such expert opinion is typically used as the basis for writing clinical guidelines. But after patients were engaged in a standardised conversation about treatment options and outcomes, only 8–15 per cent of them indicated that they wanted the surgery (Hawker *et al* 2001).

Although these studies focused on particular conditions, not health care as a whole, the role of patient preference extends well beyond elective surgery. Long-term conditions now absorb a rapidly increasing proportion of health care expenditures, and the best treatments depend greatly on patient preferences.

Consider an obese patient who presents with early symptoms of type 2 diabetes. To achieve needed weight loss, clinicians tend to recommend a slew of behaviour changes. In fact, the NHS's Quality and Outcomes Framework (QOF) evaluates clinicians based on whether they are closely monitoring no fewer than nine aspects of the disease, from HbA1c measurement to foot examinations (Khunti *et al* 2007).

To ask patients to take action to control so many distinct aspects of disease is to act in ignorance of a critically constrained resource: a patient's motivation and discipline to act. The fact that patients often face multiple long-term conditions simultaneously makes it all the more necessary to expend this resource carefully. Doctors must prioritise, based on both the potential medical benefit and on patient preferences.

For example, if the patient is eager to diet but has never been enthusiastic about exercise, the doctor should focus on what might be accomplished through dietary changes rather than demanding both dieting and exercise. Early diagnosis of patient preferences could prevent disease or escalation of disease, avoiding hospital admissions as well as major surgeries and expenses later.

Doctors do not understand the outcomes that patients prefer

The second category of evidence does not measure treatment choices directly but rather the intended outcomes from treatment. Of course, the two are closely related; a doctor is unlikely to make an accurate preference diagnosis unless he or she first understands how the patient rates various possible outcomes.

For example, before recommending a joint replacement operation instead of physical therapy, a doctor should try to assess how the patient views the implicit trade-off. Would the patient prefer chronic low-level pain moderated by routine physical therapy sessions? Or sharply reduced joint discomfort over the long term, but only after enduring a difficult and painful recovery, with possible complications? Not all patients will value the possible outcomes equally.

Several studies have documented substantial gaps between the outcomes patients prefer and the outcomes doctors *think* patients prefer.

- *Breast cancer.* As mentioned in the introduction, doctors believe that 71 per cent of patients with breast cancer rate keeping their breast as a top priority. But what is the actual figure reported by patients? 7 per cent. Furthermore, doctors believe that 96 per cent of patients scheduled to undergo chemotherapy rate living as long as possible as a top priority. Again, what is the actual figure reported by patients? 59 per cent. Finally, not one doctor reported that they believed avoiding a prosthesis was important to patients considering breast reconstruction; but 35 per cent of patients disagreed (Lee *et al* 2010).

- *Atrial fibrillation.* Many elderly patients suffering from this condition are far more wary than doctors imagine of taking blood thinners like warfarin. They worry about the potential of a difficult-to-stop bleed (Man-Son-Hing *et al* 2005).

- *Dementia.* A study of patients who faced the future prospect of end-stage dementia showed that they placed less value than doctors believed on the continuation of life with severely declining cerebral function. Through an advanced care planning process, 22 per cent of patients preferred less intensive interventions after being prompted to carefully consider what they valued (Volandes *et al* 2009).

- *Advanced cancers.* When patients with advanced cancers viewed a short video that prompted them to contemplate how they valued outcomes from life-sustaining treatments, 10 per cent and 13 per cent more preferred to avoid cardiac resuscitation and ventilation, respectively (Volandes *et al* 2012).

In addition, a large set of studies by the James Lind Foundation has shown differences between what patients value and what medical researchers prioritise (James Lind Alliance 2012). Finally, a compelling study established major differences between what doctors advise for patients and what doctors choose for themselves when they become patients, suggesting that doctors struggle to see medicine from a patient's perspective until they become patients themselves (Ubel *et al* 2011).

We believe that the government should fund many more studies in these first two categories to establish direct evidence of preference misdiagnoses across a wider array of health conditions. To date, funding for studies to understand what patients want has been limited, especially compared with the billions of pounds that are spent worldwide to research new, cutting-edge therapies, most of which deliver comparatively small marginal benefits. Given that a patient can suffer just as much from a preference misdiagnosis as from a medical misdiagnosis, a shift in funding is overdue.

There are enormous variations in care across geographic regions

The final category of evidence is the most voluminous and well documented. Decades of research have demonstrated remarkable differences in the per capita quantity of care delivered across geographic regions.

This evidence, however, is also indirect. A brief preliminary exercise helps put the data on geographic variation in perspective, by showing when a variation in care implies a preference misdiagnosis. The exercise focuses on variations in individual care, not geographic care. We will make the connection between individual and geographic variations later.

Evaluating variations in individual care
Consider the following hypothetical situation:

> *Two patients are medically identical. They have identical health states and identical diagnoses. However, they do not go to the same doctor, and they do not receive the same treatment. Is this a problem?*

What makes this exercise interesting is the wide range of possible responses. Your reaction to the question depends quite heavily on the particulars of the health state that you contemplate. We focus here on the three general narratives that guide almost all responses.

Story 1: One of the patients did not receive the proper treatment, which is clearly a problem.
You may have imagined a health state that has a definitive, well-understood, and effective treatment. Perhaps, for example, you imagined a bacterial infection that is well known to be quickly and easily cured by the right antibiotic.

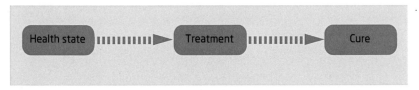

In such a case, the analysis is straightforward. One patient received the proper care and one did not. Perhaps one of the patients did not have access to care, for example. Whatever the underlying cause, if you value equity in health care, then you certainly see this as a problem.

Story 2: The doctors differed on which is the best treatment.
You may also have imagined a more complicated storyline – one in which there was more than one possible treatment, but no option that was clearly the best.

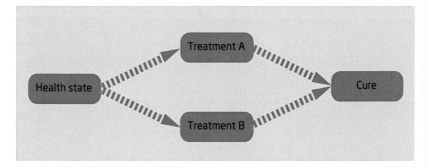

Medical evidence is often incomplete, especially for new treatments. Two doctors, exercising their experienced and independent judgement as medical professionals, could quite reasonably disagree about how best to interpret the available evidence. They could, therefore, differ in the courses of action they choose to pursue. If this is the scenario you imagined, then in all likelihood you feel that the difference in treatment is acceptable – at least temporarily, until more complete evidence is collected; or even permanently, if good evidence shows that the two treatments are equally effective.

Story 3: The patients had different treatment preferences.
Finally, you may have imagined a scenario in which it was unclear which of several possible *outcomes* was preferable. Notice that in the first two storylines the outcome was unambiguous and obviously desirable: 'cure'. If only real medicine were so simple!

The reality is that most medical treatments involve choices and trade-offs. Most treatments have both positive and negative outcomes. Quite frequently, for example, there is a trade-off between quality of life and life expectancy. A major surgery or medical regimen such as chemotherapy might increase life expectancy but leave a patient facing a difficult recovery and coping with troublesome side effects for the rest of his or her life.

Therefore, disagreement on whether the benefit of a particular treatment outweighs the harm is reasonable and commonplace. In the diagram below, some people might prefer outcome A, while others prefer outcome B. (Note that by 'outcome' we are referring to a composite of positive and negative results – typically, of therapeutic benefits and side effects. Note also that one of the treatment options may be not to treat at all.)

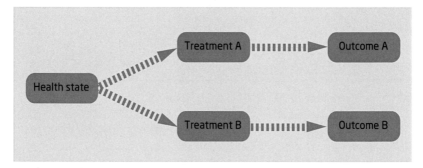

If this is the scenario you imagined, then you may not have perceived there to be a problem. You may have imagined that each patient received the treatment that he or she preferred.

But this, as it turns out, is too happy a story. A more likely narrative is that neither patient had the information they needed to evaluate which outcome they preferred. And, unfortunately, the doctors did a poor job of diagnosing what either patient *would* want were they fully informed. Instead, they were guided by other influences.

If it worked out that both patients received the treatment they would have preferred had they been fully informed, then this was probably a matter of luck. The more likely and unhappy outcome is that one or both patients suffered the consequences of a preference misdiagnosis.

A summary of explanations for variations in individual care

Remember that our intention with this exercise was to make a connection between a *variation in care* and a *preference misdiagnosis*. The connection is hardly automatic. A preference misdiagnosis, in fact, is just one possibility. The variation between medically identical patients could be explained by:

- a failure to deliver the right treatment (or, sometimes, the right non-treatment)

- a difference between doctors regarding *what treatments do*

- a difference between doctors regarding *what patients want*, which could be:
  - an accurately diagnosed difference in the patients' preferences
  - a preference misdiagnosis.[2]

Note that in the first explanation above, the patients and doctors all agreed on the right thing to do; there was simply a failure to execute. In the second, doctors and patients all agreed on the desired outcome, but not on the right treatment to reach

2 It could also be a combination of more than one of these factors, but this possibility will not affect our analysis.

that outcome. (They agreed on the *end*, but not on the *means to the end*.) In the third, there were differences in the desired outcomes, either between patients or between patients and their doctors.

With these possibilities in mind, let's turn to the data on geographic variation.

From individual variation to geographic variation

For decades, a team of researchers based in the United States at Dartmouth, led by John Wennberg, has extensively documented stunning variations in the utilisation of care in the United States – not from patient to patient, but from geographic region to geographic region (Wennberg and Gittelsohn 1973; Dartmouth Atlas of Health Care 2012; Wennberg 2010). These variations are so significant that the team often expresses the differences not in percentage terms but in multiples.

These variations are hardly unique to the United States though. In fact, they were first discovered and described in England and Wales by J Alison Glover, who reported *tenfold* variation in the incidence of tonsillectomies (Glover 1938). Variations in care of similar magnitude persist to this day (Department of Health 2011), and have been reported in many other countries in an increasing number of studies (Wennberg International Collaborative 2012).

The evidence is clear and undisputed. Nobody has cast any doubt on the fact that there are enormous differences in the consumption of health care services from one region to the next. The more interesting question is: Why? Let's return to the hypothetical exercise above. We have to make one change as the unit of analysis shifts from individual patients to regions.

Recall that the premise in the hypothetical exercise was two medically identical patients. Of course, no two geographic regions are medically identical. There may be variations that depend on demographic variables such as age, income level, and race, plus variations tied to other variables such as predominant occupations, climate, and more. Furthermore, one region might suffer from an outbreak of an infectious disease or could be accidentally exposed to an acute environmental toxin. Therefore, we must now consider a fifth possible source of variation – variation in aggregate health states.

Recapping, variation in care between two geographic regions can be explained by:

■ failures to deliver treatments known to be effective

■ differences between doctors regarding what treatments do

■ differences between doctors regarding what patients want, which could be:
  ■ accurately diagnosed differences in patient preferences
  ■ preference misdiagnoses

- differences in aggregate health states.

It is very difficult to precisely quantify each of these five sources. However, our intent is not to make a precise calculation; it is only to show that the silent misdiagnosis is an enormous problem. Therefore, we can simplify the analysis by making some reasonable conjectures about the relative magnitude of the five sources of variation. We argue that three of the five sources are so small relative to the total observed variation that they are of little consequence. Let's look at each of these three factors.

Geographic variation in delivery of treatments known to be effective. This category of care includes treatments for which there is virtually universal agreement that the treatment is effective; for example, the use of clot-busting medication and aspirin in the immediate aftermath of a heart attack.

Unfortunately, even where there is near-universal agreement, there is still some variation. The magnitude of this variation, however, is much smaller than the geographic variation in health care as a whole. Furthermore, only about 15 per cent of health care spending falls into this category (Wennberg 2010). These variations are worthy of vigorous response, but they represent only the tip of the variation iceberg.

Geographic variation in patient preferences. There is a paucity of research that has explored the extent to which patient preferences vary with geography. However, while we know that variations can be dramatic from one *patient* to the next, why would we expect to find variation from one *geographic region* to the next?

On the one hand, it is not hard to pick a few specific treatments for which preferences might reasonably vary with geography. For example, it would not be surprising to find a very high preference for cosmetic surgery in Hollywood.

Considering health care in aggregate, however, it is simply not plausible to imagine that patients, if fully informed, might prefer much more health care in some locations than in others. In the United States, Medicare recipients in Miami consume three times as much health care per capita as Medicare recipients in Minneapolis. The variations are no less dramatic in the UK, where per capita expenditures for care of patients with cancer or musculoskeletal, circulatory or respiratory problems vary twofold to threefold among NHS primary care trusts (PCTs) (Department of Health 2010). Certainly, this cannot be because residents of Miami or other high-utilisation regions thoroughly enjoy the experience of visiting GPs, being referred to specialists or for tests, or lying sick in a hospital bed being poked and prodded by strangers.

In fact, in the absence of data showing dramatic geographic variations in patient preferences, we can reasonably hypothesise that they are small when compared with other sources of variation. This hypothesis is supported by two studies. One concluded that there was little regional variation in preference for seeing specialists or having tests (Anthony *et al* 2009). Another study did show a significant regional variation in preference for joint replacement surgery, but the magnitude of that variation was dwarfed by the difference between what patients wanted and what doctors *thought* they should want (Hawker *et al* 2001).

Geographic variation in health states. The line of argument is similar here. While there are certainly variations in health states from one geographic region to another, it is implausible to imagine that the very large observed variations in care could be explained by geographic variations in aggregate health states. Are Medicare recipients in Miami really so much sicker than those in Minneapolis that they require three times the total per capita spending on health care? Certainly, the variations in health states are far less than that.

Some health care leaders have defended the high utilisation of care in their home regions by claiming that their patients *really are* that much sicker. To prove their case, they have even calculated risk adjustments based on the number of diagnosed conditions among patients in their region. The problem with this line of argument is that high-utilisation regions spend more not just on treatments, but also on diagnostics. This can produce more diagnoses per person in high-utilisation regions than for medically identical persons in low-utilisation regions. The additional diagnostic labels skew the risk adjustments and make the population look sicker than populations who have not undergone the same intensity of testing (Song *et al* 2010; Welch *et al* 2011).

The table below summarises the analysis so far.

Table 1 Sources of geographic variations in care

Geographic variation in delivery of care known to be effective	SMALL
Plus geographic variation created by doctors differing on what treatments do	
Plus geographic variation created by accurate preference diagnoses	SMALL
Plus geographic variation due to preference misdiagnoses	
Plus geographic variation in aggregate health states	SMALL
TOTAL OBSERVED GEOGRAPHIC VARIATION IN CARE	VERY LARGE

Thus, we can see that the total variation (V_{TOT}) is approximately equal to the sum of the variation due to doctors' differing beliefs regarding what treatments do ($V_{DD\text{-}WTD}$), plus the variation due to preference misdiagnoses (V_{PM}):

$$V_{TOT} \approx V_{DD\text{-}WTD} + V_{PM}$$

So, the next obvious question is: which of the two remaining factors, $V_{DD\text{-}WTD}$ and V_{PM}, account for the bulk of V_{TOT}?

As a first step, it is important to recognise that a reasonable initial instinct is that *both* $V_{DD\text{-}WTD}$ *and* V_{PM} must be small numbers, following a similar logic we used to discuss geographic variations in patient preferences and aggregate health states. While there is nothing unusual or surprising about two *individual* doctors taking a different view of the outcome of a treatment or the outcome a patient would prefer, how could two *geographic regions* be in strong disagreement? Why wouldn't there be a diversity of opinion within each region? Why wouldn't the average for each region be near the average for the nation as a whole?

Of course, doctors in a given region influence each other through social and professional interactions, and it is reasonable to expect some degree of homogenisation within regions as a result. This effect, however, hardly seems forceful enough to account for the dramatic variations that are actually observed. If we are to believe that $V_{DD\text{-}WTD}$ and V_{PM} are large numbers, then we must develop a stronger hypothesis about why. What forces could be powerful enough to affect the *collective* medical judgement of an entire geographic region?

Counterintuitive as it may seem, there *are* such forces. The Dartmouth analysis has shown that there is a very strong connection between consumption of health care in a geographic region and the availability of health care resources. It is *not* the case, for example, that the residents of Minneapolis have the same number of hospital beds, imaging machines, doctors, and community nurses, per capita, as the residents of Miami, and utilise them only one-third as often. Minneapolis has fewer resources, which are distributed differently.

Could the mere presence of available resources affect decisions about the treatment that patients receive? Could it affect preference diagnoses? Many doctors recoil at the suggestion because, quite naturally, they want to believe that they are scientific, unbiased, and patient-centred in their decision-making.

Doctors, however, are not Spock-like computing machines, and we should not expect them to be. They are human, and their judgement in the face of uncertainty is affected by numerous factors other than the patient's health state and preferences.

It is not hard to see how the presence of available resources could be a powerful force. First, all other things being equal, when facing a serious health condition and uncertainty, patients and doctors alike prefer action to inaction. Both instinctively find it far more comfortable to do everything possible to fight disease than to simply watch and wait.

This bias for action is reinforced by the reality that doctors, like all people, have selective memory. Many doctors will find it hard to ever forget the patient who died following a decision *not* to treat. However, they may never again think of a patient they *did* treat to no clear benefit. They may even rationalise a treatment's serious side effects in the belief that the treatment probably saved the patient's life.

The mere presence of available resources also makes it more likely that doctors will consume those resources 'just to be safe'. They will keep patients in the hospital just a little bit longer. They will order more tests just to be absolutely certain that they haven't missed anything. They may even lower the diagnostic threshold at which they consider treatment appropriate. They will do all of this just to be prudent.

These are powerful explanations, but there are still more. For example, the media is a powerful force that raises patients' expectations. With increasing frequency, patients arrive at the doctor's door with the belief that they deserve – in fact, they are entitled to – the best that medicine has to offer. They may insist upon treatment while unaware of potential negative consequences that may outweigh the benefits. When facing such demands, if resources are available, and if the treatment is a reasonable choice given the uncertainties, even a doctor who would not advise the treatment based on his or her independent and unbiased medical judgement may find it much more practical to satisfy the patient than deny them. The possibility of a legal entanglement only reinforces this bias. Judges and juries tend to find action a more persuasive defence than inaction.

Finally, doctors have a bias for action because they prefer to stay busy. Most are attracted to the profession for altruistic reasons – to help patients. The intuitive connection between being busy and having greater impact is natural. There are, of course, less altruistic reasons why doctors may have a bias for staying busy. In the United States, compensation is usually tied to the quantity of services delivered. Even in the UK, where such direct ties are much less common, doctors may naturally and understandably fear that if they, or colleagues in their specialty, are not busy, their services may no longer be required.

In summary, then, there are plenty of plausible reasons to believe what at first seems an unlikely conjecture: that the collective judgement of a group of doctors can be influenced by factors that have nothing to do with patients' medical conditions or preferences. These factors are tied to the availability of resources in a given region. Note that two categories of uncertainty – in either *what treatments do* or in *what patients want* – are equally able to open decision making to these influences.

Let's now return to our approximation:

$$V_{TOT} \approx V_{DD\text{-}WTD} + V_{PM}$$

We now have reason to believe that both $V_{DD\text{-}WTD}$ and V_{PM} might be very large numbers. Unfortunately, given the research and the data available today, we cannot calculate how much each source of variation contributes to the total. We certainly *should* be able to do so. Indeed, the fact that we cannot represents a tremendous gap in knowledge that must be filled.

That said, our argument is simply that V_{PM} is a large number, and that preference misdiagnoses are, therefore, rampant within the NHS. Whether the silent misdiagnosis accounts for 20 per cent, 40 per cent, 60 per cent or 80 per cent of total variation is quite irrelevant. At any of these levels, the silent misdiagnosis represents a gross injustice to patients – not to mention an opportunity for the NHS to save billions of pounds while simultaneously serving patients better.

We would argue, in fact, that if another researcher wishes to defend the counterhypothesis that the incidence of the silent misdiagnosis is trivially small, the burden of proof rests squarely and heavily upon his or her shoulders. To make the case, that researcher would have to show that each of the studies in the first two categories we described was anomalous or an exception to the rule. Furthermore, that researcher would naturally seek a persuasive piece of evidence in the geographic data itself. Specifically, they would try to show that as medical evidence for treatments for a particular health condition accumulate, V_{TOT} declines to near zero.

Bear in mind that V_{DD-WTD} is created when doctors have different views regarding what treatments do. These differences are enabled by scientific uncertainty. As such, as evidence from medical studies accumulates, V_{DD-WTD} should decline. In fact, *if V_{PM} were trivially small*, we'd expect V_{DD-WTD} *and* V_{TOT} to steadily decline to near zero as evidence accumulates. However, among treatments for which patients clearly have different preferences when fully informed, we are unaware of any that exhibit almost no geographic variation.

Furthermore, if V_{PM} were trivially small, then we'd expect to find decreases in V_{TOT} over time after major new studies were released. But geographic variation proves stubborn in the face of evidence accumulated over years and even decades. The NHS Atlas shows nearly fivefold variation in hysterectomy and nearly fourfold variation in knee replacement, for example. Furthermore, in the five years since the publication, in 2006, of a well-known study on disc herniation, the decline in geographic variation in procedures for disc herniation has been modest (Weinstein *et al* 2006; Department of Health 2011). And since the publication of the COURAGE (Clinical Outcomes Utilizing Revascularization and Aggressive Drug Evaluation) trial in 2007, which showed that percutaneous intervention for stable coronary disease failed to reduce rates of death or heart attack any more than optimal medical therapy, variation continued unabated. Nearly tenfold differences were observed among the 152 PCTs in England in 2010 (Boden *et al* 2007).

Taken together, the three categories of evidence presented here strongly suggest that preference misdiagnoses are rampant. Nobody should be surprised by this. Doctors are simply not taught that making a preference diagnosis is important, or that preference diagnoses, like medical diagnoses, can be challenging.

Unaware of what patients would want if they were fully informed, and believing that patients expect an expert recommendation, doctors either insert their own values or are swayed by the availability of resources that surround them. They make their treatment decisions without sufficient insight into patient preferences, and then simply assert that what they have chosen is what patients should want. Unfortunately, doctors are rarely, if ever, confronted with evidence to show they are wrong in this assertion.

As such, there are people in every corner of the UK who, like Susan, suffer preference misdiagnoses. They suffer as unnecessarily and as dramatically as patients who, like Linda, suffer a medical misdiagnosis. And yet, their stories are silent.

First steps to a solution

We have already stated that our central recommendation is to implement an NHS-wide measure of the accuracy of preference diagnoses. Even with such a measure, however, there will be little chance of success unless the NHS also tackles a handful of erroneous assumptions about how health care works.

Tackling five erroneous assumptions

There are at least five assumptions that are in direct conflict with the mindset necessary to stop the silent misdiagnosis.

Stop believing that science alone determines need

Too many of the policy-makers who shape health care systems around the world suffer from a single collective delusion – that the 'right answers' in health care are strictly a matter of science. This assumption can, of course, also be convenient for doctors and patients. It allows doctors to believe that they are the experts who decide the proper treatment, and it allows patients to believe simply that 'doctor knows best'. That way, they do not have to take responsibility for decision-making, or live with the regret of having made a decision that led to a bad outcome.

However, the reality is that science is but one determinant of the proper treatment. A patient's preferences matter just as much.

Stop believing that variation is the problem

For too long, the NHS and other health services around the world have acted as though variation, in and of itself, is the big problem that must be addressed. That view is problematic.

Geographic variation is an intriguing and unsettling observation, but is not, in and of itself, a problem. The silent misdiagnosis is a problem; the lack of outcomes research, and the medical uncertainty that it creates, is a problem; but variation is not. In fact, we should be pleased to see variation wherever it matches variations in health states or patient preferences.

Nonetheless, the received message in the NHS and in other health policy circles around the world has been simply to 'reduce variation'. If that is the objective, the solution is simple: gather data on the outcomes that treatments produce and then use the data to establish specific treatment guidelines, standardising medicine to the greatest extent possible. Witness, for example, how the NHS has, for the past decade and more, invested heavily in gathering evidence and publishing guidance through the National Institute for Health and Clinical Excellence (NICE).

This could be a very successful approach in driving out variation that is rooted in scientific uncertainty. Unfortunately, it would simultaneously exacerbate the problem of the silent misdiagnosis. Two patients who present identical health states *should not* always be given the same treatment. Medicine must be made sensitive to the values of individual patients. Otherwise, the silent misdiagnosis will persist.

In theory, if the NHS were to standardise medicine, it would slash *geographic* variation in care to almost zero. It is important to recognise, however, that doing so would *not* stop the silent misdiagnosis. We used evidence of geographic variation to support our case that the silent misdiagnosis is an enormous problem. It is *not* the case, however, that zero geographic variation implies zero silent misdiagnoses.

Standardisation of medicine would simply push the variation created by preference misdiagnoses from the regional level to the individual level. Under a regime of standardised medicine, for example, *all* breast cancer patients might receive lumpectomy with radiation therapy instead of a mastectomy, even though a significant subset of women would choose mastectomy were they fully informed.

The NHS is currently wrestling with the ethics of standardisation in its policy for breast cancer screening. A policy that all women receive mammograms starting at age 50 or younger may well save lives. However, recent studies have documented a high incidence of over-diagnosis of breast cancer and the unnecessary surgeries it leads to (Cancer Research UK 2012; Welch and Schwartz 2011). Screening can bring real benefits but also real harms and, were they fully informed, women would have different preferences. The choice is not one for policy-makers, but one for individual patients. Standardisation *guarantees* preference misdiagnoses.

Stop believing that patient choice is about time and location

The NHS has expended enormous energy on making care more patient-centred. Early in 2002, for example, the then Secretary of State for Health, Alan Milburn, made a firm commitment to patient choice (Department of Health 2002). At first, the objective clearly included giving patients a stronger voice in choosing their treatments. But that proved difficult, and within just a few years the focus shifted to giving patients greater control over *where* and *when* they were treated.

In 2004, for example, a Department of Health directive, Choose and Book, instructed PCTs to provide patients with four to five hospital choices, particularly for procedures that had long waiting times; but it was silent on the question of treatment choice (Department of Health 2004). The following year's directive described new approaches for engaging patients, but still focused far more heavily on the time and place of treatment (Department of Health 2005). This pattern has continued (Le Grand 2009). Imagine how customers would react if McDonald's restaurant gave its customers the power to choose which restaurant they ate at and when, but insisted that what they ate would be chosen by its in-house culinary experts! Unless this mindset is challenged, patients will continue to be harmed by the silent misdiagnosis.

Stop believing that 'the market' can sort out health care

Markets may be the most powerful tool ever devised for organising economic activity, rooting out inefficiencies, and stimulating innovation. But markets are also an imperfect tool, and particularly so in health care. This is not to say that markets and health care should never meet, but it certainly means that markets should be applied to health care with caution.

This is hardly new thinking. In a seminal article published in the 1960s, Stanford economist and Nobel Laureate Kenneth Arrow discussed how the market model could be adapted for health care (Arrow 1963). Critically, he imagined that doctors needed to act as professional agents for their patients, deciding on their behalf what treatment was best. But this led him to consider another pressing question – what behavioural expectations should we have of doctors, given that patients entrust them with life and limb? Arrow recognised that the extraordinarily high expectations were reasonable, given the circumstances. Indeed, he advocated for extensive training and licensing of physicians.

The medicine that Arrow imagined, however, was overwhelmingly science-driven, not preference-driven. We now understand that this view is flawed. Preferences matter. Doctors will never be effective professional agents unless they are able to accurately diagnose patient preferences. Therefore, if we are to cling to Arrow's notion of an internal market guided by professional agents, we must also impose an unforgiving behavioural expectation on our doctors: they must aspire, with energy and enthusiasm, to the ideal of making an accurate preference diagnosis for each and every patient.

Enthoven went further (Enthoven 1985). He advocated a curriculum for doctors that extended well beyond medicine to management, including course work in microeconomics, finance, accounting, marketing, organisational behaviour, and decision science. Following a similar line of thinking, in 2011, Dartmouth College launched a new Master of Health Care Delivery Science programme, which brings together the faculties of medicine, business, and arts and sciences. the Mayo Clinic will offer a similar degree in collaboration with Arizona State University in 2013. Not every doctor needs such training, but it is certainly appropriate for those with responsibility for the quality and efficiency of service delivery for large populations.

Stop believing that commissioners can calculate need

Commissioners are the lynchpin in the NHS's internal market. They are the key figures on the demand side of the equation. Each commissioner contracts with suppliers – hospitals, clinics, and the like – to provide the quantity of resources that he or she assesses is necessary for his or her geographic region.

It sounds like a straightforward job, but there is one small problem. How can commissioners possibly know the proper quantity of resources to provide? They have little choice but to base their calculations heavily on measures of the existing system – either in their own region, or in other regions, or even from other parts of the world. And the only problem with that is that *all* such data are severely compromised by the silent misdiagnosis. The data reflect the many biases that impair doctors' decision-making in the face of scientific uncertainty and ignorance about what patients want. Little, if any of it, reflects what patients would demand were they fully informed.

As a result, commissioners struggle and, in the absence of a better mechanism for assessing what patients would prefer were they fully informed, they will always struggle. Whether they are organised into 152 PCTs or more than 500 clinical commissioning groups, whether they do their own work or rely extensively on consultants, whether they have completed PhDs, medical degrees, or merely survived university, they will struggle. Without a reliable signal of true demand, the commissioner's job is rather akin to being dropped into an uncertain location, miles from where you need to be but enshrouded in dense fog, all the while knowing that every time you take more than a tiny step in any direction at all, you'll anger someone with political clout.

As a result, we should not be surprised to find that there are such dramatic variations in the supply and consumption of health care from one region to the next. Without good diagnostics of patient preferences, commissioning is simply an impossible job, doctors cannot be effective professional agents, and the internal market is unworkable.

This is not a happy situation, especially given the long-term consequences of commissioning decisions. Thanks to the many biases that affect doctors in their decision-making, built hospital beds are filled beds, purchased imaging machines are fully utilised imaging machines, and pockets of excess supply can persist for decades – sometimes leaving other needs *under*-resourced.[3] And wherever there is a mismatch between supply and true demand, the silent misdiagnosis looms large.

---

3 In 1959, the economist Milton Roemer was asked about the wisdom of the Hill-Burton Act, passed in 1946, the same year that parliament authorised the NHS. The Hill-Burton Act was a far less ambitious attempt to improve health equity by building hospital beds to reach a standard level of 4.5 beds per 1000 population. His reply that 'a built bed is a filled bed' became known as Roemer's Law, which is frequently used to describe the correlation between capacity and utilisation in health care (Roemer 1961).

Measure and report the accuracy of preference diagnoses

Tackling these five erroneous beliefs, throughout the NHS, would pave the way for powerful change. Guiding that change would be a single statistic – a measure of the accuracy of preference diagnoses. Bearing in mind the timeless management maxim, 'measure something and it will improve', by far the most important step the NHS must take to stop the silent misdiagnosis is to measure and report the accuracy of preference diagnoses.

Several researchers have already shown that such a measure is possible. They have designed experiments that assess how dramatically treatment choices change after patients become well informed (*see* earlier section, 'The evidence'). These assessments must exit the realm of research and enter the realm of daily operations within the NHS.

The mechanics of such a measure are conceptually straightforward. A small but statistically meaningful subset of patients, randomly selected, would be asked to participate. Timing is important; the request would have to come immediately after a treatment decision but before treatment begins. If a patient agreed, they would receive a layperson's 'crash course' in the medical evidence regarding the possible harms and benefits of each of their treatment options. Researchers have devised a range of sophisticated patient decision aids that could be used or modified for this purpose (Elwyn *et al* 2010; Stacey *et al* 2011). The patient's understanding would be checked, and their level of knowledge documented.

Finally, they would be asked a simple question: *Have you changed your mind?* If they have, then the doctor initially involved in the treatment decision made a preference misdiagnosis (in this case, happily, one that could be corrected before treatment). The incidence of preference misdiagnoses can then be calculated and reported, and the NHS's progress in stopping the silent misdiagnosis tracked.

More critically, doctors could be given immediate feedback when they make such errors. The best among them would have sufficient intrinsic motivation to attack preference misdiagnoses with intense self-reflection. The best hospitals would invest the same level of interest and energy in discussing preference errors as the profession currently brings to other clinical issues, such as unexpected deaths or serious adverse events. Over time, error rates would decline.

The courts could add extra force to the effort to improve the accuracy of preference diagnoses. English law on informed consent is based on the premise that the doctor selects the treatment and the patient consents to or refuses the doctor's recommendation. The doctor, however, is not required by law to provide information about alternative treatment options. As a result, the door remains wide open for a preference misdiagnosis. By contrast, a few systems in the United States, including the Group Health Cooperative of Puget Sound, a health maintenance organisation governed by its patients, made great strides in reducing preference misdiagnoses *after* legislators set a more demanding legal standard – one that requires documentation to show that patients have a clear understanding of their options and likely outcomes.

Implementing a measure of the incidence of preference misdiagnoses would, however, require a new investment in information systems. It would also require the co-operation of doctors, who would need to initiate the measurement process just as a treatment decision is made. That said, the systems adopted by PCTs to support and manage referrals made by GPs, including referral management centres, could be redirected and augmented for just this purpose (Imison and Naylor 2010).

Towards a more complete solution

While measurement and reporting is the most important step, more needs to be done. In particular, the full burden of stopping the silent misdiagnosis must not rest on the shoulders of doctors. Doctors can and must spend more time talking with patients about what they want – that is, diagnosing their preferences. But these conversations are not enough. Doctors need help to diagnose patient preferences; they need better information, and they need their patients to have better information. The reason that the silent misdiagnosis is so prevalent is that doctors and patients make decisions behind a veil of ignorance. Doctors know far too little about what patients want, and patients know far too little about the treatment options, outcomes, and evidence for the condition they have.

Greater access to information would bring us closer to the textbook model of an ideal market. In fact, it would stop the silent misdiagnosis overnight, as patients would simply announce which treatment they preferred. We are, of course, nowhere near this idealised state today, and practical constraints will prevent us from ever reaching it.

Nonetheless, we need to push toward the ideal, by working both sides of the problem, as suggested by Figure 1 below. We must make both patients and doctors better informed.

Figure 1 The risk of silent misdiagnosis is related to both clinician and patient knowledge

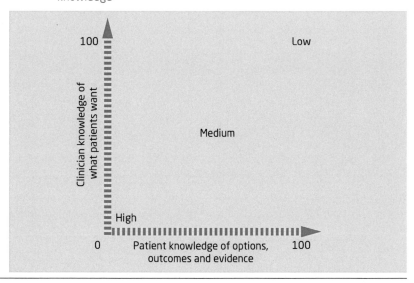

But what is the best way to deliver such information to doctors and patients? It is hardly a trivial challenge, as several innovators have discovered in their endeavours to inform patients more fully using patient decision aids.

In the early 1990s, the Informed Medical Decisions Foundation produced one of the most sophisticated patient decision aids ever (Morgan *et al* 2000).[4] Focusing on stable coronary heart disease, the Foundation built a highly interactive computer-based resource with information tailored to patients' specific clinical circumstances. The architects of the decision aid even added predictive models that helped patients envision the consequences of their choices, in the short term and long term. With carefully framed information that avoided unintended biases, the decision aid helped patients understand, for example, that surgery can both increase long-term survival rates and lower short-term survival rates (thanks to potential complications from the surgery). Based on such information, a patient whose biggest remaining hope in life was to attend his daughter's wedding six months hence might choose to forgo the surgery.

The designers of this decision aid knew that patients would struggle to assess how they might feel in the future about health states that they had not yet experienced. So they videotaped conversations with other patients who had already lived through various treatments and outcomes. The tool even generated printouts intended to facilitate productive follow-on conversations between patients and their caregivers – conversations that made it easy for patients to clearly express their preferences.

However, patients do not always find it easy to form a preference and make a choice they feel confident in. Preferences are constructed slowly, through a process of becoming informed, thinking through options, and deliberating with others. The role of the decision aid is to help support this process.

Because decision aids have proven powerful (Stacey *et al* 2011) for those who have actually used them, their designers are understandably frustrated that their actual use in clinical practice is quite limited. Research into barriers that inhibit the adoption of decision aids has been revealing (Gravel *et al* 2006; Coulter and Collins 2011; Coulter 2011). Efforts to increase the accuracy of preference diagnoses will face a number of practical constraints, including:

■ doctors' busy schedules

■ some doctors' willingness to involve patients in decision-making

---

4 The effort proceeded in collaboration with an international team based at Duke University and with funding from Kaiser Permanente and the US Agency for Health Care Policy and Research, now the Agency for Healthcare Research and Quality (AHRQ).

- some doctors' lack of trust in the information contained in decision aids, particularly whether the information is up to date, unbiased, and tailored to local conditions

- some patients' willingness to take greater responsibility for their own care

- some patients' willingness to invest time and energy learning about treatment options and outcomes

- some patients' ability to think rationally and carefully, especially when sick or scared

- some patients' ability to absorb information that includes at least some degree of medical and statistical complexity

- some patients' ability to evaluate how they feel about potential outcomes that they have never experienced

- the necessary funding to build sophisticated decision aids and keep them up to date and locally relevant.

These are real and challenging practical constraints. Nonetheless, the NHS should strive for perfection. It should build sophisticated decision aids for more health conditions and then find ways to break through the constraints.

That said, the NHS must not let the perfect become the enemy of the good. We are far enough from perfection that any step in the right direction would be welcome. Therefore, the NHS should look to make progress with a full range of possibilities that lie between doing nothing and implementing highly sophisticated decision aids.

Indeed, there are many possibilities. It is not our intention to make a specific prescription, but rather to lay out a range of options. The most sensible solution will probably vary according to the context; for example, long-term versus episodic care, diagnostic versus screening tests, medicine versus surgery, and crisis versus non-crisis care.

Provide information that improves doctors' ability to diagnose preferences

We should not be surprised by the fact that the silent misdiagnosis is so prevalent. Some basic information that would make doctors better informed is either unavailable or not widely disseminated and studied.

Provide aggregate data on outcome preferences

The most basic information that all doctors should demand is data that describe *aggregate preferences for populations*. As we noted earlier, there are enormous gaps between the outcomes that patients value and those that doctors *think* they value. If doctors simply had access to, and studied, basic statistics that describe aggregate outcome preferences, they could start with a much more informed estimate of what an individual patient preferred – even before meeting the patient for the first time.

In fact, given the life-and-limb responsibilities that we entrust to doctors, shouldn't we demand that they are well educated in the outcomes that the average patient values? For example, shouldn't more doctors who treat breast cancer be aware that only 7 per cent of breast cancer patients rate keeping their breast as one of their top three priorities? Moreover, aren't facts like these as fundamental to the practice of effective medicine as facts like 'the thigh bone is connected to the hip bone'?

Unfortunately, we know of no broad-based database of patients' outcome preferences. We only know of the studies of selected individual conditions described in the section entitled 'The evidence'(*see* pp 13–14).

While aggregate data on outcome preferences would be valuable in the effort to stop the silent misdiagnosis, doctors must interpret such data with caution. In particular, they must recognise that the value patients place on various outcomes is just one of three dimensions of outcome preferences. To see why, consider two patients who place identical value on each of the relevant outcomes for a given treatment. These two patients might not choose the same treatment were they fully informed, for one of two reasons. First, not all patients will have the same attitude towards risk. One patient, for example, might be willing to accept a 1 per cent risk of death during surgery to achieve a desirable therapeutic outcome, while the other would never take such a risk. Second, not all patients place the same importance on short-term and long-term outcomes. One patient might be far more willing than another, for example, to endure short-term pain to achieve long-term gain.

Provide aggregate data on treatment preferences

Aggregate data about treatment preferences is potentially more desirable than aggregate data about outcome preferences. It is more direct and more actionable. And it can, in theory, capture all three dimensions of outcome preferences: the value placed on outcomes, risk attitudes, and time trade-offs.

However, such data must be gathered more carefully, with the assistance of sophisticated patient decision aids. While a modestly informed patient can express an outcome preference, only a well-informed patient can express a treatment preference that is a reliable indication of what a similar patient might want were they fully informed.

Provide data on the general health preferences of individuals

While population aggregates are useful, nobody would be pleased with a system in which all patients are treated as 'average'. Doctors must be wary of any natural inclination to stereotype. While aggregate statistics are useful, they must only be used to support first approximations. Each patient must then be respected as an individual, and their individual preferences diagnosed.

Out of respect for each patient's uniqueness, doctors should demand measures of variation, such as standard deviation, for certain indicators of aggregate outcome preferences. Where variation is high, doctors should recognise the need to be much more thoughtful about how an individual patient varies from the population mean. And they should be even more eager to ascertain any patient-specific information that helps them to make that assessment.

One possibility is that the NHS could develop a survey-based instrument that assessed *general* as opposed to *disease-specific* patient preferences. As part of routine check-ups, patients could fill out a questionnaire that reveals general health preferences on any number of dimensions, including (but certainly not limited to) quality of life versus length of life, live for the moment versus live for the future, how my body looks versus how my body functions, and averse to experimental therapies versus eager to try them.

We view such questionnaires as at least loosely analogous to personality tests. Patients could even have a four-letter 'preference profile' similar to the Myers-Briggs personality type. A simple, four-letter code at the top of each patient's health record could offer doctors quick guidance on how the preferences of the patient in front of them vary from average preferences for the population. The mere presence of such questionnaires and codes would serve as a reminder to doctors and patients alike that individual patient preferences are important.

To our knowledge, no such questionnaire has ever been developed for this purpose. This is an untested idea. However, such instruments are routinely used in business to develop differentiated offerings for customer groups with distinct needs.

Though untested, such an instrument could help doctors make better preference diagnoses. There is no reason why doctors must start each preference diagnosis from scratch, assuming nothing. When a red-faced overweight man in his 50s walks into the emergency department complaining of chest pain, doctors are much more likely to focus on a medical diagnosis of coronary heart disease than they would if the patient were an athletic-looking woman in her 20s. The patient's appearance does not make the medical diagnosis, but it helps form an initial hypothesis to be verified through further information-gathering. A general health preference profile could play a similar role for preference diagnoses.

That said, were such an instrument used to help doctors diagnose patient preference, it would be crucial to recognise that health preferences are likely to be less stable than personalities. Professional financial advisers know that it is important to periodically reassess an individual client's life goals and risk profile, especially following major life events such as marriage, the birth of a child, or a job change. Similarly, general health preferences would need to be reassessed every few years and following significant life-changing events. They cannot be regarded as *traits*, but rather as *states* that change as life changes (Mulley 1989).

Of particular note, it is quite possible that the experience of illness itself might alter a patient's general health preferences. Until more is known about this possibility, doctors should interpret general preference profiles cautiously. They can be used to shape initial hypotheses, but not as conclusive instruments. Doctors could use them to start conversations with patients. For example: 'Your profile indicates that you are quite averse to surgery. How do you feel about that, now that you know that the symptoms you have would very likely be ameliorated by surgery?'

Note that aggregate preferences for populations and general health preferences for individuals could be combined to provide doctors with even more useful data. Aggregate statistics could be reported for population subsets with the same general health preferences. The aggregate data could also be analysed by standard demographic groupings such as age group or income level. Such analysis might guide doctors to make a comment like the following to a patient: 'Research shows that among well-informed patients that are similar to you – roughly your age and strongly prioritising quality of life over longevity – only 3 per cent choose prostatectomy to reduce the risk of death from cancer. Does that surprise you? Before deciding, would you like to view a video of patients who *did* choose prostatectomy describing its after-effects?'

Measure progress

In addition to providing doctors with more information about what patients want, the NHS must also assess whether doctors are using it and learning from it. This could be achieved through simple testing of doctors as part of their annual performance appraisals. Qualitative assessments of how hard doctors are working to improve preference diagnoses should also be part of these appraisals.

Provide information that helps patients express what they want

As we have said, the gold standard is a well-informed patient who expresses their preference clearly and directly. This is, of course, not always attainable. A 'crash course' in a disease, its treatment options, outcomes, and evidence takes time and energy from both the patient and the health system. Doctors are tightly scheduled, and many patients also have time constraints. Some patients may also lack the necessary cognitive capabilities.

Therefore, it makes sense to pursue practical solutions that respect these real-world constraints. Even a little bit of information can be extremely valuable. For example, one research study examined how patients eligible for a prostate-specific antigen (PSA) test responded after spending roughly 15 minutes with a video and brief discussion that presented information on three topics: the basics about the natural progression of prostate disease, the accuracy of the PSA test, and the effectiveness of treatments for prostate cancer. After receiving the information, the proportion of patients who could accurately answer basic questions on these three topics rose dramatically, from an initial range of 10–40 per cent, depending on the question, to 70–90 per cent. More critically, this information had a huge impact: the proportion of patients choosing to be screened dropped from 98 per cent to 50 per cent (Frosch *et al* 2001).

While these results are impressive, quick decision aids such as these must be designed with care. Several studies have shown that the way information is framed can have a dramatic impact on how patients react. For example, the two statements 'There is a 97 per cent chance that you will survive this surgery' and 'There is a 3 per cent chance that you will die during this surgery' are mathematically identical, but patients react very differently to them.

Inform patients during the doctor-patient interaction

The time patients and doctors have face-to-face is particularly scarce. Indeed, doctors frequently report that they do not use sophisticated decision aids because they do not fit easily into their available time or existing work processes.

One possible response is to make the decision aids simple and quick. This is the philosophy behind the use of option grids – one-page tables that compare treatment options and answer questions frequently asked by patients (Option Grid Collaborative 2012; Lloyd *et al* 2012). They are designed to facilitate conversations that can take place in the few minutes available during clinical visits. They at least partially inform patients and point them in the right direction should they want more information.

Inform patients outside of the doctor's office

Given how much patients need to learn in order to make an informed choice, the NHS must also work to inform patients outside of the context of the patient–doctor interaction. Not all knowledge needs to be transferred from the mouth of a doctor to the ear of the patient. Well-trained health care assistants, nurses, or health coaches, working in a high-performing team with doctors, could also guide patients through options. Alternatively, well-designed decision aids are nearly completely self-guided.

Inform patients in advance

Finally, if scarcity of time is one of the primary practical barriers to patients becoming well informed, why not start early? Some treatment decisions can be anticipated months in advance – for example, decisions related to childbirth.

Another good example is screening. We know that patients may reasonably disagree, for example, on whether or not they wish to have a mammogram to screen for breast cancer. The NHS encourages such tests starting at the age of 50, and there is a move toward screening women younger than 50. There is a trade-off for patients, however. Mammograms can lead to over-diagnosis, which has only recently been recognised as a potential harm of the screening. Instead of just prompting women to report for the test when they reach the eligible age, why not prompt them a year earlier that they will need to make a decision soon about whether they want mammograms, and point them towards a useful decision aid?

Unfortunately, the current system attempts to elicit preferences in advance for only one aspect of medicine: end-of-life care. Asking patients to state preferences for every imaginable disease state in advance is obviously impractical. However, when patients are at high risk of a particular disease, or face degenerative diseases with predictable progressions, why wait for the actual medical diagnosis?

Measure progress

The NHS ought to measure how much patients know when making health decisions. Several researchers are already working on ways to do this. In particular, they have proposed measures of *decision quality* that include assessments of how well patients are informed (Sepucha *et al* 2004; Scholl *et al* 2011; Sepucha *et al* 2008). Most assessments are carried out at the critical point when a treatment decision is made. Patients are, quite literally, tested on their knowledge of their own disease, their treatment options, and the probable outcomes.

This, we believe, is the most essential aspect of decision quality, but some of the measures proposed go further. Some assess how confident a patient is in their treatment decision and how ready they are to proceed with treatment. Others assess how meaningfully a patient was involved in choosing a treatment. And some compare outcome preferences to treatments to determine how closely these are aligned.

Any of these measures of decision quality could be aggregated to assess the performance of clinics, hospitals, or geographic regions. Indeed, if hospitals were to compete on measures of decision quality – such as how well they inform patients and how well they match treatments to patients' preferences – it would almost certainly accelerate the elimination of the silent misdiagnosis (Sepucha and Mulley 2009).

We have made a number of recommendations that imply substantial investments in information technology, such as:

- measuring the incidence of preference misdiagnoses
- measuring how much patients know about their disease and their treatment options
- measuring how much doctors know about what patients want
- collecting aggregate information about patient preferences
- building patient decision aids that include outcomes as described by patients who have already grappled with the disease.

Such systems may seem far-reaching and far removed from what exists today. But some initiatives are already under way in two specialised clinics within the Dartmouth-Hitchcock Medical Center – its Comprehensive Breast Program and Spine Center. In fact, Dartmouth has now entered into a joint effort known as the High Value Health Care Collaborative to create a national database. Fifteen other institutions are involved, including the Cleveland Clinic, Denver Health, Intermountain Healthcare and the Mayo Clinic. The NHS could inspire a similar collaboration among its leading health care institutions and clinical commissioning groups to capture patient-reported measures, including outcome and treatment preferences.

From ideas to action

Today, patient preferences are a very weak force in driving treatment decisions. The good news is that there is greater opportunity now to tackle this problem than there has been for decades.

Under the 2012 Health and Social Care Act, the UK government has charged the NHS Commissioning Board with the task of making the principle of shared decision-making the norm in the NHS. The vision is that patients are better informed and more engaged in choosing their treatments, confident that there will be 'no decision about me without me' (Coulter and Collins 2011).

In this paper, we have advocated for this and more. Yes, stopping the silent misdiagnosis will require patients who are better informed about their options – but it will also require doctors who are better informed about what patients want. In addition, it will require changing the mindset throughout the NHS, elevating the urgency of stopping the silent misdiagnosis and tackling the deeply embedded assumptions that have let this situation continue. Finally, and most critically, the NHS must measure, publish, and publicise data on the accuracy of preference diagnoses.

It is one thing to define this agenda, but quite another to make it happen. In recent years, there have been significant advances in the field of *innovation execution,* which focuses on identifying the best practices for making innovation happen inside of established organisations (Govindarajan and Trimble 2010). One insight from this field is the critical importance of distinguishing between a *change agenda* and an *innovation agenda.*

The objective of a change programme is to bring about a specific and definitively desirable change in thinking and behaviour *throughout an organisation.* The objective of an innovation initiative, by contrast, is to execute a new and uncertain project *without doing any harm to ongoing operations.* Change is imperative; but innovation is experimental. Change is about altering what exists; innovation leaves what exists untouched and unharmed, while simultaneously testing a new possibility on the side.

The agenda that we have proposed includes both change and innovation, as follows.

Change agenda
- Tackle the five entrenched but flawed assumptions that stand in the way of stopping the silent misdiagnosis. We described the five assumptions in 'First steps to a solution', (*see* pp 25–8.)

- Measure and report the accuracy of preference diagnoses.

Innovation agenda
- Find ways to better inform patients about treatment options, outcomes, and evidence.

- Find ways to better inform doctors about what well-informed patients want.

While there is little doubt that it would be a good thing to have better-informed patients and better-informed doctors, what is quite uncertain is how to go about making them better informed. There are several possibilities, as we described above, but there is no way of knowing in advance which would be most successful. In fact, it is not even clear whether giving patients better information or giving doctors better information would lead to a faster and more powerful result. Thus, these items are for the innovation agenda, not the change agenda.

How to execute change

There are multiple models for change (Kotter 1996), but most agree that the proper next steps include the following:

- establishing a sense of urgency through a strong leadership narrative that communicates why stopping the silent misdiagnosis is so important

- creating a powerful coalition of 'true believers' who constantly reinforce the message

- empowering employees to act, and, in particular, encouraging doctors to shift a significant fraction of their time and energy from medical diagnosis to preference diagnosis

- measuring and reporting progress

- holding every employee, at all levels, accountable for stopping the silent misdiagnosis.

The last two steps are particularly critical. Right now, two metrics that get close attention in many hospitals and in doctor performance reviews are the incidence of patient complaints and the length of waiting lists. Of course, these are relevant metrics. But ensuring that each patient gets the treatment they would choose were they fully informed is equally critical, if not more so. Therefore, a reported measure of the accuracy of preference diagnoses must be prominent on scorecards at every level in the NHS – scorecards for policy-makers, commissioners, medical directors, and individual doctors.

How to execute innovation

Models for executing innovation start with the simple premise that an innovation initiative is a *project* that requires additional work for an organisation. These models focus first on the physics of getting the work done; but one of the biggest challenges here is the simple reality that employees are already extremely busy. They have full-time jobs, with little slack in their schedules.

Step one in innovation execution is to divide the labour into two categories – tasks that can easily fit into the workflows of existing employees (with, at most, a bit of training) and tasks that do not. For tasks that fit existing workflows, if available slack time is inadequate, it may be necessary to *expand the staff* to make it reasonable to expect employees to do both their existing jobs *plus* the new project work. Then, to tackle the tasks in the latter category, it is necessary to commission *dedicated teams* – that is, teams composed of employees who are assigned full-time, or very nearly full-time, to the innovation initiative.

Consider, for example, one of the approaches to informing patients described above: the option grid. As a very rough approximation, the option grid strategy requires two tasks: creating and updating option grids, and discussing them with patients. The first task does not fit easily into any existing workflows in the NHS, and thus requires the creation of a dedicated team. The second task – discussing the option grids with patients – naturally fits into existing patient– doctor consultations. However, we shouldn't assume there is sufficient slack time in doctors' schedules, even though option grids are designed to be discussed in roughly three minutes. Unless there is a way to easily cut three minutes from what doctors are already discussing with patients, scheduled appointments must be lengthened, if only by a few minutes. In areas where schedules are already filled to maximum capacity, recruiting more staff must be considered.

Such a move is painful when resources are tight. However, there is no way to make innovation happen on the cheap, and the downstream benefits of stopping the silent misdiagnosis are enormous.

Creating special teams to lead change and innovation

We have described several approaches to providing better information to doctors (about what patients want) and to patients (about options, evidence, and outcomes). All would require dedicated teams to implement.

One dedicated team could focus on gathering data about aggregate preferences for particular conditions, another on developing surveys that elicit general patient preferences, a third on devising option grids, and a fourth on building more complete patient decision aids. Though the NHS could certainly create one or more new sub-units to house these dedicated teams, another option is to identify existing organisations whose functions could be redirected or augmented to take on these tasks. For example, we've already suggested that re-purposed referral management schemes might be well positioned to gather data on aggregate preferences at the time of decision-making. The NHS Information Centre might provide co-ordination and expertise based on its experience with patient-reported outcome measures (PROMs). In addition, decision aids are already being developed by the NHS and in academic collaboratives (NHS Rightcare).

There may also be a role for NICE. Few organisations have had so powerful an impact on the role of evidence-based health care in the UK. Furthermore, the task of gathering and disseminating information on *what patients want* is quite analogous to the task of gathering and disseminating information on *what treatments do,* which NICE publishes in the form of evidence-based guidance for clinical practice.

One method for gathering data on what patients want is to survey patients at just the right time, as they are actively contemplating treatment decisions. Modestly informed patients could offer information as to how they prioritise their goals; well-informed patients could indicate specific treatment preferences.

Further, this process of gathering preference data could be the first step in what have been called comprehensive cohort trials or 'preference trials'. The first steps would be to inform patients using sophisticated decision aids, elicit their preference, and gather aggregate preference data. Patients who preferred one treatment or the other would get that treatment. Patients who were indifferent between the two treatments could be randomised in the traditional manner for clinical trials. Outcomes for all patients would be measured. Such preference trials could be at the heart of the NHS's process for organisational learning, providing continuously improved knowledge of what works for whom and what is valued by whom.

A valid concern about this approach is that only patients who are indifferent about the treatment options are randomised. However, there are at least three offsetting benefits. First, giving patients choice in their treatment and randomising only those who are at personal equipoise is a more ethical approach to clinical trials. Second, if this approach were widely used, it would be possible to directly measure the extent to which outcomes are better when patients choose their own treatment (McPherson *et al* 1997). Finally, patients could report whether actually experiencing the treatment caused them to reconsider how they valued various outcomes. Such data would be valuable to future patients. For example, women who have opted for post-mastectomy breast reconstruction surgery have often been disappointed by the result. Future patients should be aware of this phenomenon before choosing a treatment.

While this approach may be unfamiliar to many, it is not hypothetical. The Spine Patient Outcomes Research Trial (SPORT) (Weinstein *et al* 2006) at Dartmouth used exactly this design and also invested heavily in the patient-reported outcome measures most useful to patients trying to assess their own treatment goals. This led to the aforementioned High Value Health Care Collaborative, which is creating a national database to improve preference diagnosis and care delivery.

A new game for commissioners

We do not imagine that commissioners are well positioned to gather and distribute information to patients and doctors. Their focus will continue to be on the allocation of scarce resources within their geographic regions – across the full breadth of services, from community-based mental health services to paediatrics and more.

What commissioners need to understand, however, is that providing better information to patients and doctors will have a dramatic impact on the quantity of services demanded. Today, this quantity is distorted by the silent misdiagnosis. Eliminate that distortion and the result will be significant – perhaps even double-digit – changes, as true demand is revealed. Some service lines will see increases; even more will see decreases. As projected in the 2002 Wanless Report, engaged patients will work with clinicians, co-managing their care delivery and co-producing better health.

Over the coming months, the newly formed clinical commissioning groups will need to prioritise continuity of services. They will need to sustain business as usual and ensure that no significant gaps in care arise as a result of the 2012 Act and its organisational changes. Looking over a longer time horizon, however, commissioners will need to shift their focus to smoothly navigate the changes in demand that will come about as a result of the elimination of silent misdiagnoses. To do so, commissioners will have to understand that historical demand will become an ever less relevant guide to future demand.

To anticipate the direction in which demand is heading, commissioners should pay close attention to any new data about what well-informed patients want. Indeed, they must assign greater importance to information about what well-informed patients want than to other, higher-volume signals. For example, patient advocacy groups may be vocal, but they sometimes represent minority interests.

Most data about what well-informed patients want will consist of national averages. While such information will be a good indicator of true demand in a region for most conditions, some preferences may vary by region, and commissioners must try to be attentive to these variations to estimate true demand in their particular region.

As we have said, true demand is the quantity of services that would be demanded were the silent misdiagnosis stopped. To estimate how long it will take to reach true demand, commissioners need to track the trend in the incidence of silent misdiagnoses. As the incidence is reduced, actual demand will move towards true demand.

Of course, stopping the silent misdiagnosis will not be easy, and may take many years. In the interim, commissioners can consider how to nudge if not push the system in the right direction. Consider, for example, elective percutaneous intervention (PCI) for stable coronary artery disease. In 2010, the rate of provision in 152 PCTs varied from just more than 10 to just fewer than 100 per 100,000 people per year. If there were newly published national data adjusted for age and gender and other factors which showed that well-informed patients preferred PCI over optimal medical therapy at a rate of 50 per 100,000, commissioners should contemplate whether it makes sense to accelerate the move towards true demand.

For example, they could closely examine the incidence of preference misdiagnoses for that particular treatment in their high- or low-rate region. Also, the commissioners might ask, is there any reason to believe that well-informed patients would, on average, prefer more or less PCI in my region than nationally? If preference misdiagnoses were high and there was no reason to believe that the region had an unusually high or unusually low true demand, the commissioner could consider proactively reallocating resources to adjust the capacity for PCI. As mismatch of supply and demand is, in and of itself, a contributor to the silent misdiagnosis, such a move would help stop it.

To be clear, what we are proposing is that commissioners play an entirely new game – one guided by true demand as revealed through a vigilant effort to stop the silent misdiagnosis. Commissioners can no longer be guided by politics, by outcries over waiting lists, or by spending comparisons with other European countries. Such pressures led the UK to ramp up its investment in health care from 6 per cent to 9 per cent of gross domestic product (GDP) during the years of investment through the *NHS Plan*. Unfortunately, these investments, like those before and since, were made in the absence of clear insights into what patients would want if they were fully informed. As a result, the NHS may well have over-invested in capacity to provide some treatments while it under-invested in capacity to provide services that would provide greater value to patients. Commissioners must play a new game.

Conclusion

The silent misdiagnosis is a widespread problem in the NHS. While a preference misdiagnosis may be less obvious than a medical misdiagnosis, the consequences for the patient can be just as severe.

The NHS must break this silence. It must do so by measuring and tracking the incidence of preference misdiagnoses. It must also help doctors to avoid these errors by providing them with tools and information that will help them make better inferences about what patients want. Finally, it must provide patients with tools and information that help them understand treatment options, outcomes, and evidence, so that they are better able to articulate their preferences to doctors. As doctors and patients become more informed, the incidence of the silent misdiagnosis will subside, and true demand will be revealed.

Putting an end to the silent misdiagnosis would bring many benefits: patients would get the health care they truly want; the public would benefit as public expenditure on health care was redirected to other sectors where it is badly needed; and health professionals would achieve both reduced pressures for operational efficiency and the elevated satisfaction that comes with being confident that they are delivering the right care, every time, to every patient.

References

Anthony DL, Herndon MB, Gallagher PM, Barnato AE, Bynum JPW, Gottlieb DJ, Fisher ES, Skinner JS (2009). 'How much do patients' preferences contribute to resource use?'. *Health Affairs*, vol 28, no 3, pp 864–73.

Arrow K (1963). 'Uncertainty and the welfare economics of medical care'. *American Economic Review*, vol 53, pp 941–73.

Barry MJ, Cherkin DC, Chang Y, Fowler FJ, Skates S (1997). 'A randomized trial of a multimedia shared decision-making program for men facing a treatment decision for benign prostatic hyperplasia'. *Disease Management and Clinical Outcomes*, vol 1, no 1, pp 5–14.

Boden WE, O'Rourke RA, Teo KK, Hartigan PM, Maron DJ, Kostuk WJ, Knudtson M, Dada M, Casperson P, Harris CL, Chaitman BR, Shaw L, Gosselin G, Nawaz S, Title LM, Gau G, Blaustein AS, Booth DC, Bates ER, Spertus JA, Berman DS, Mancini GB, Weintraub WS, COURAGE Trial Research Group (2007). 'Optimal medical therapy with or without PCI for stable coronary disease'. *New England Journal of Medicine*, vol 356, no 15, pp 1503–16. doi:10.1056/NEJMoa070829

Cancer Research UK (forthcoming). *Breast Screening Review*. Chaired by Sir Michael Marmot.

Coulter A (2011). *Engaging Patients in Healthcare*. New York: Open University Press.

Coulter A, Collins PA (2011). *Making Shared Decision-Making a Reality: No decision about me, without me*. London: The King's Fund.

Dartmouth Atlas of Health Care (2012). 'Understanding of the efficiency and effectiveness of the health care system'. Dartmouth Atlas website. Available at: www.dartmouthatlas.org (accessed on 30 April 2012).

Department of Health (2011). *The NHS Atlas of Variation in Healthcare: Reducing unwarranted variation to increase value and improve quality* [online]. Right Care website. Available at: www.rightcare.nhs.uk/index.php/atlas/atlas-of-variation-2011/ (accessed on 3 May 2012).

Department of Health (2010). *The NHS Atlas of Variation in Healthcare: Reducing unwarranted variation to increase value and improve quality* [online]. Right Care website. Available at: www.rightcare.nhs.uk/index.php/atlas/atlas-of-variation-2010/ (accessed on 3 May 2012).

Department of Health (2005). *Creating a Patient-Led NHS: Delivering the NHS Improvement Plan*. London: Department of Health.

Department of Health (2004). *Choose & Book: Patient's choice of hospital and booked appointment*. London: Department of Health.

Department of Health (2002). *Delivering the NHS Plan: Next steps on investment, next steps on reform*. Cm 5503. London: HMSO.

Deyo RA, Cherkin DC, Weinstein J, Howe J, Ciol M, Mulley AG, Jr (2000). 'Involving patients in clinical decisions: impact of an interactive video program on use of back surgery'. *Medical Care*, vol 38, no 9, pp 959–69.

Eddy D (1994). 'Principles for making difficult decisions in difficult times'. *Journal of the American Medical Association*, vol 271, no 22, pp 1792–8.

Elwyn G, Tilbert J, Montori V (2012). 'The ethical imperative for shared decision making'. *Journal of Evaluation of Clinical Practice* (in press).

Elwyn G, Frosch D, Volandes AE, Edwards A, Montori VM (2010). 'Investing in deliberation: a definition and classification of decision support interventions for people facing difficult health decisions'. *Medical Decision Making*, vol 30, no 6, pp 701–11. doi:10.1177/0272989X10386231

Enthoven A (1985). *Reflections on the Management of the National Health Service: An American looks at incentives to efficiency in health services management in the UK*. London: Nuffield Provincial Hospitals Trust.

Frosch D, Kaplan R, Felitti V (2001). 'The evaluation of two methods to facilitate shared decision making for men considering the prostate-specific antigen test'. *Journal of General Internal Medicine*, vol 16, no 6, pp 391–8.

Glover JA (1938). 'The incidence of tonsillectomy in school children: (section of epidemiology and state medicine)'. *Proceedings of the Royal Society of Medicine*, vol 31, no 10, pp 1219–36.

Govindarajan V, Trimble C (2010). *The Other Side of Innovation: Solving the execution challenge*. Boston: Harvard Business School Press.

Gravel K, Légaré F, Graham I (2006). 'Barriers and facilitators to implementing shared decision-making in clinical practice: a systematic review of health professionals' perceptions'. *Implementation Science*, vol 1, no 16.

Hawker GA, Wright JG, Coyte PC, Williams JI, Harvey B, Glazier R, Wilkins A, Badley EM (2001). 'Determining the need for hip and knee arthroplasty: the role of clinical severity and patients' preferences'. *Medical Care*, vol 39, no 3, pp 206–16.

Imison C, Naylor C (2010). *Referral Management: Lessons for success*. London: The King's Fund.

James Lind Alliance (2012). 'Tackling treatment uncertainties together'. Lind Alliance website. Available at: www.lindalliance.org (accessed on 17 April 2012).

Kennedy A, Sculpher M, Coulter A, Dwyer N, Rees M, Abrams K, Horsley S, Cowley D, Kidson C, Kirwin C, Naish C, Stirrat G (2002). 'Effects of decision aids for menorrhagia on treatment choices, health outcomes, and costs: a randomized controlled trial'. *Journal of the American Medical Association*, vol 288, no 21, pp 2701–8.

Khunti K, Gadsby R, Millett C, Majeed A, Davies M (2007). 'Quality of diabetes care in the UK: comparison of published quality-of-care reports with results of the Quality and Outcomes Framework for Diabetes'. *Diabetic Medicine*, vol 24, no 12, pp 1436–41. doi:10.1111/j.1464-5491.2007.02276.x

Kotter J (1996). *Leading Change*. Boston: Harvard Business School Press.

Le Grand J (2009). 'Choice and competition in publicly funded health care'. *Health Economics, Policy and Law*, vol 4, issue 4, pp 479–88. doi:10.1017/S1744133109990077

Lee CN, Dominik R, Levin CA, Barry MJ, Cosenza C, O'Connor AM, Mulley AG Jr, Sepucha KR (2010). 'Development of instruments to measure the quality of breast cancer treatment decisions'. *Health Expectations*, vol 13, no 3, pp 258–72. doi:10.1111/j.1369-7625.2010.00600.x

Lloyd A, Joseph Williams N, Beasley A, Tomkinson A, Elwyn G (2012). 'Shared decision making in a multidisciplinary head and neck cancer team: a case study of developing Option Grids'. *International Journal of Person Centered Medicine* (in press).

Man-Son-Hing M, Gage B, Montgomery A, Howitt A, Thomson R, Devereaux PJ, Protheroe J, Fahey T, Armstrong D, Laupacis A (2005). 'Preference-based antithrombotic therapy in atrial fibrillation: implications for clinical decision making'. *Medical Decision Making*, vol 25, no 5, pp 548–59.

McPherson K, Britton AR, Wennberg JE (1997). 'Are randomized controlled trials controlled? Patient preferences and unblind trials'. *Journal of the Royal Society of Medicine*, vol 90, no 12, pp 652–6.

Morgan MW, Deber RB, Llewellyn-Thomas HA, Gladstone P, Cusimano RJ, O'Rourke K, Tomlinson G, Detsky AS (2000). 'Randomized, controlled trial of on interactive videodisc decision aid for patients with ischemic heart disease'. *Journal of General Internal Medicine*, vol 15, no 10, pp 685–93.

Mulley A (1989). 'Assessing patients' utilities. Can the ends justify the means?'. *Medical Care*, vol 27, vol 3, suppl, S269–81.

Murray E, Davis H, Tai SS, Coulter A, Gray A, Haines A (2001). 'Randomised controlled trial of an interactive multimedia decision aid on benign prostatic hypertrophy in primary'. *British Medical Journal*, vol 323, pp 493–9.

NHS Rightcare website. Available at: www.rightcare.nhs.uk (accessed on 8 May 2012).

Option Grid Collaborative (2012). 'Option grid'. Option Grid website. Available at: www.optiongrid.co.uk (accessed 30 April 2012).

Roemer M (1961). 'Bed supply and hospital utilization: a natural experiment'. *Hospitals*, vol 35, pp 36–42.

Rothberg MB, Sivalingam SK, Ashraf J, Visintainer P, Joelson J, Kleppel R, Vallurupalli N, Schweiger MJ (2010). 'Patients' and cardiologists' perceptions of the benefits of percutaneous coronary intervention for stable coronary disease'. *Annals of Internal Medicine*, vol 153, no 5, pp 307–13. doi:10.1059/0003-4819-153-5-201009070-00005

Scholl I, van Loon MK, Sepucha K, Elwyn G, Légaré F, Härter M, Dirmaier J (2011). 'Measurement of shared decision making – a review of instruments'. *Zeitschrift für Evidenz, Fortbildung und Qualität im Gesundheitswesen*, vol 105, no 4, pp 313–24.

Sepucha KR, Mulley AG (2009). 'A perspective on the patient's role in treatment decisions'. *Medical Care Research and Review*, vol 66, no 1, suppl 53S–74S. doi:10.1177/1077558708325511

Sepucha KR, Levin C, Uzogara E, Barry M, O'Connor A, Mulley A (2008). 'Developing instruments to measure the quality of decisions: early results for a set of symptom-driven decisions'. *Patient Education and Counseling*, vol 73, no 3, pp 504–10.

Sepucha KR, Fowler J, Mulley A (2004). 'Policy support for patient-centered care: the need for measurable improvements in decision quality'. *Health Affairs*, suppl vari, VAR54–62.

Song Y, Skinner J, Bynum J, Sutherland J, Wennberg JE, Fisher ES (2010). 'Regional variations in diagnostic practices'. *New England Journal of Medicine*, vol 363, no 1, pp 45–53. doi:10.1056/NEJMsa0910881

Stacey D, Bennett C, Barry M, Col N, Eden K, Holmes-Rovner M, Llewellyn-Thomas H, Lyddiatt A, Légaré F, Thomson Rl (2011). 'Decision aids for people facing health treatment or screening decisions'. *Cochrane Database of Systematic*

Reviews, as well as issue 10, article CD001431. doi:10.1002/14651858.CD001431. pub3.

Ubel PA, Angott AM, Zikmund-Fisher BJ (2011). 'Physicians recommend different treatments for patients than they would choose for themselves'. *Archives of Internal Medicine*, vol 171, no 7, pp 630–4. doi:10.1001/archinternmed.2011.91

Volandes AE, Levin TT, Slovin S, Carvajal RD, O'Reilly EM, Keohan ML, Theodoulou M, Dickler M, Gerecitano JF, Morris M, Epstein AS, Naka-Blackstone A, Walker-Corkery ES, Chang Y, Noy A (2012). 'Augmenting advance care planning in poor prognosis cancer with a video decision aid: a preintervention-postintervention study'. *Cancer*. Advance online publication. doi:10.1002/cncr.27423

Volandes AE, Paasche-Orlow MK, Barry MJ, Gillick MR, Minaker KL, Chang Y, Cook EF, Abbo ED, El-Jawahri A, Mitchell SL (2009). 'Video decision support tool for advance care planning in dementia: randomised controlled trial'. *British Medical Journal*, vol 338, b2159.

Wagner E, Barrett P, Barry M, Barlow W, Fowler F (1995). 'The effect of a shared decisionmaking program on rates of surgery for benign prostatic hyperplasia'. *Medical Care*, vol 33, no 8, pp 765–70.

Wanless D (2002). *Securing our Future Health: Taking a long-term view. Final report.* London: Department of Health.

Weingart SN, Wilson RM, Gibberd RW, Harrison B (2000). 'Epidemiology of medical error'. *British Medical Journal*, vol 320, no 7237, pp 774–7. doi:10.1136/bmj.320.7237.774

Weinstein JN, Tosteson TD, Lurie JD, Tosteson AN, Hanscom B, Skinner JS, Abdu WA, Hilibrand AS, Boden SD, Deyo RA (2006). 'Surgical vs nonoperative treatment for lumbar disk herniation – the Spine Patient Outcomes Research Trial (SPORT): a randomized trial'. *Journal of the American Medical Association*, vol 296, no 20, pp 2441–50.

Welch H, Schwartz L (2011). *Overdiagnosed: Making people sick in the pursuit of health.* Boston: Beacon Press.

Welch HG, Sharp SM, Gottlieb DJ, Skinner JS, Wennberg JE (2011). 'Geographic variation in diagnosis frequency and risk of death among Medicare beneficiaries'. *Journal of the American Medical Association*, vol 305, no 11, pp 1113–8. doi:10.1001/jama.2011.307

Wennberg DE, Marr A, Lang L, O, Malley S, Bennett G. 'A randomised trial of a helpline care management strategy'. New England Journal of Medicine 2010, vol 363, no 13, pp 1245–55.

Wennberg JE (2010). *Tracking Medicine: A researcher's quest to understand health care*. Oxford: Oxford University Press.

Wennberg JE (2004). 'Practice variation: implications for our health care system'. *Managed Care*, vol 13, no 9, suppl, pp 3–7.

Wennberg J, Gittelsohn A (1973). 'Small area variations in health care delivery'. *Science*, vol 182, pp 1102–18.

Wennberg International Collaborative website. Available at: www. wennbergcollaborative.org/ (accessed on 30 April 2012).